ADVANCE PRAISE

"Dr. Stillman is that rare caring, compassionate, and competent physician. His book on autoimmunity is an easy, insightful, and enjoyable read. Since autoimmunity is increasingly common and commonly misunderstood, his book is timely. Do yourself a favor and read it now. For you and those you love, this synthesis is needed. Well written and well documented, it is a refreshing understanding on a commonly misunderstood condition. As a pioneer in integrative and functional care, it is a pleasure to highly recommend this contribution."

—Russ Jaffe, MD, PhD, Founder and Chief Executive Officer of PERQUE Integrative Health, LLC

"Autoimmune disease used to be a rare occurrence when I began practicing medicine. Not so anymore. Nearly 5 percent of the US population has been diagnosed with an autoimmune disease. And that number is much higher as it takes most physicians a long time period to begin checking their sick patients for autoimmune disease.

"Leland Stillman, MD, is trying to reverse this trend. His book The End of Autoimmunity should be read by all physicians who are treat-

ing patients, as well as anyone else interested in how to optimize their health. This book provides up-to-date information on how to properly diagnose and treat an autoimmune disorder by looking for an underlying cause. Conventional medicine does not look for underlying causes of autoimmune illnesses. Once diagnosed, patients are treated in a cookie-cutter manner using toxic drug therapies that disrupt immune function.

"Dr. Stillman describes a holistic approach, searching for toxicities—including aluminum, mercury, electromagnetic pollution, drugs, vaccines, and 'sick building syndrome'—as well as dietary imbalances. Identifying these underlying causes and using a holistic protocol to accelerate and promote healing has proven successful for Dr. Stillman's patients.

"I have been practicing medicine for over three decades. I have utilized an approach similar to Dr. Stillman's in treating my autoimmune patients. I have also found good success with my patients. This is an important book that addresses autoimmune disease. I highly recommend my colleagues and anyone interested in a rational approach to medicine read this book."

—David Brownstein, MD, author of seventeen books, including *Iodine: Why You Need It, Why You Can't Live Without It*, www.drbrownstein.com

"Most physicians managing autoimmune disease are treating the smoke while ignoring the fire. Dr. Stillman goes after the fire—and this book shows exactly how he does it."

—Ben Greenfield, *New York Times* bestselling author of *Boundless*

"Medicine advances when physicians are willing to publish what they see, even when it disrupts consensus. The End of Autoimmunity is a direct challenge to a system that has grown comfortable managing decline. Dr. Stillman is not merely questioning protocols; he is questioning first principles. Why are autoimmune diseases accelerating? Why are we suppressing immune systems instead of restoring them? This is not a theoretical book, and it is not timid. It is a clinician's account of documented recoveries achieved by addressing root causes. It will unsettle the complacent—and empower the serious."

—Simone Gold, MD, JD, Founder of America's Frontline Doctors and CEO of GoldCare.com

"I highly recommend The End of Autoimmunity. At a time when autoimmune disease is skyrocketing and patients are told their only option is lifelong immunosuppression, Dr. Stillman has the courage to challenge the status quo. This book exposes the environmental and medical blind spots driving chronic illness and backs it up with real clinical cases. Whether you agree or disagree with every point, it will force you to think differently about the autoimmune epidemic."

—Dr. Ben Tapper, DC

"In The End of Autoimmunity, Dr. Stillman transforms the journey of complex disease into a peaceful path toward healing, and he provides empowering tools that will help people get well. For many struggling with an autoimmune illness, this may be the only book you need to find health."

—Derek Guillory, MD

"We need more doctors like Leland who are willing to actually think instead of mindlessly doing the bidding of the pharmaceutical industry. He makes the necessary effort to seek upstream causes and real solutions to complex chronic illnesses."

—Ty Vincent, MD

"A central idea since ancient times is that the body must rest, recuperate, and cleanse from the metabolic activity that keeps us vital and energetic. Autoimmune disease describes a situation where fire, or inflammation, outpaces the ability of our bodies to repair and cleanse, associated with water. Dr. Stillman, in a no-nonsense way you can understand, lays out the key elements of how this balance is lost and makes you sick. Part of this is confronting the toxicity of modern life as one of the drivers of inflammation. This builds a trail you can follow back toward health. Highly recommended."

—Paul K. Branch, MD, Holistic Solutions MD

"Dr. Stillman is doing what most physicians are too cautious or too comfortable to do—following the clinical evidence wherever it leads, including into territory that makes the establishment deeply uncomfortable. This book is not a polemic. It is a physician's honest accounting of what he has actually seen, what has worked, and what the conventional paradigm cannot explain and therefore refuses to acknowledge. The cases are real. The reasoning is sound. The willingness to name the problem is rare. I recommend it to every patient who has been told their labs are normal while they continue to suffer, and to every clinician who suspects the current model is failing the people it claims to serve."

—Edward Pomicter, MD, anesthesiologist turned integrative physician specializing in hormonal Optimization and Metabolic Health

"Brave, thorough, and long overdue. Dr. Stillman is a hero for speaking up, asking the hard questions, and advocating for patients in a way that medicine desperately needs."

—SALOME MASGHATI, MD, BOARD-CERTIFIED GYNECOLOGIST

"Dr. Stillman may not be your doctor, but he just might be your doctor's doctor. His methods get results. This book is the synthesis of functional medicine, environmental medicine, and quantum biology that we have needed for a long time."

—DANE MOSHER, DO

"This work presents a decisive shift away from symptom-based medicine toward a deeper understanding of environmental and physiological drivers of disease. Grounded in clinical experience, it raises important questions that modern medicine can no longer afford to ignore."

—CARLOS LOREDO RITTER, MD, PEDIATRIC NEUROLOGIST AND SLEEP MEDICINE EXPERT

"With autoimmune conditions like Hashimoto's thyroiditis on the rise, I'm seeing more and more people struggling with thyroid issues, fatigue, and symptoms that just don't make sense. In The End of Autoimmunity, Dr. Leland Stillman takes a different approach. Instead of just managing symptoms, he digs into the root cause of why the body is breaking down in the first place. If you're tired of being told everything is 'normal' when you know it's not, and you don't want another pill for your autoimmunity, this book will open your eyes to what's really going on and what you can actually do about it."

—DR. AMIE HORNAMAN, "THE THYROID FIXER"

"The End of Autoimmunity is the manual that all awake healthcare professionals have been waiting for for decades. Instead of trying to track down each bit of information on vitamin D, iodine, vitamin C, and so on, Dr. Stillman has done all of us a huge service by putting this critical information together in one place—with exact instructions concerning how to use it. Bravo, and thank you!"

—CHRISTIANE NORTHRUP, MD, *NEW YORK TIMES* BESTSELLING AUTHOR OF *GODDESSES NEVER AGE*, *THE WISDOM OF MENOPAUSE*, AND *WOMEN'S BODIES, WOMEN'S WISDOM*

"Fearless in pursuit of truth, exposing the hidden factors—including the mouth—that fuel autoimmunity."

—MATTHEW KOGAN, DMD, NMD

"Dr. Stillman has written the manual that the pharmaceutical industry hopes you never read."

—KATHLEEN HORSTMEYER, BOARD-CERTIFIED NATUROPATHIC DOCTOR

"For years, Dr. Stillman has been relentlessly researching and applying the best ways to help autoimmune patients recover. This book clearly outlines what he's learned and, most importantly, how to apply it. Dr. Stillman combines the best of traditional, functional, and quantum medicine in his framework that will shed new light for both patients and practitioners."

—MEREDITH OKE, EXECUTIVE COACH AND HOST OF THE *QUANTUM BIOLOGY COLLECTIVE* PODCAST

"A must-read for anyone looking to simplify their approach to health in a world dominated by expensive gimmicks and noise. Support your body's ability to repair, and it will heal. That's God's design!"

—TORI JENSEN, BSN, RN, RD

"In the time I have been working in holistic health, and the years I spent with Leland training mineral balancing practitioners, I have not known a more knowledgeable and curious MD. His ability to synthesize allopathic and holistic health principles into something unique and equally coherent has been a joy to watch. This ability gives him a powerful insight into the origins of autoimmunity and what to do about it."

—Clark Engelbert, Founder of Nutritional Analytics

"Current research suggests that heavy metals, industrial chemicals, and various forms of environmental pollution are major driving forces behind the rapidly increasing incidence of autoimmune diseases worldwide. While genetics create a baseline susceptibility, environmental factors are estimated to cause up to 70 percent of autoimmune cases. Dr. Stillman, in his very interesting book, further points to these and other culprits behind our epidemic of autoimmunity, including heavy metals, chemicals, and electromagnetic pollution. This is a timely book and one that everyone with autoimmunity should read."

—Olle Johansson, PhD, professor, retired (but still active) from the Karolinska Institute and the Royal Institute of Technology, both in Stockholm, Sweden

"For two decades at GreenMedInfo, I have watched the published science accumulate around aluminum toxicity, mercury burden, EMF exposure, and iatrogenic harm—while mainstream medicine continued prescribing immunosuppression and calling it care. Dr. Stillman has synthesized that evidence into a clinical framework that actually works, documented by real patients with real outcomes. This is not medical heresy. It is medicine doing what medicine is supposed to do."

—Sayer Ji, Founder of GreenMedInfo and author of *Regenerate*

"Dr. Stillman pulls back the curtain on a medical system that has traded true healing for lifelong suppression. By addressing environmental toxins and clinical blind spots, he challenges the dogmas driving the modern autoimmune epidemic. If you're tired of being told your condition is incurable, this book provides a clinical framework and evidence-based hope for real healing."

—Dr. Sina McCullough, co-host of the *Beyond Labels* podcast and author of *Hands Off My Food*

"The End of Autoimmunity is a fearless, case-backed clinical manual that names the environmental toxins and medical dogmas driving today's autoimmune epidemic, from aluminum and mercury to EMFs and chemical sunscreens. Dr. Stillman doesn't just challenge the status quo; he offers a documented path to remission, giving hope to patients who have exhausted conventional medicine. Get this book and read it from cover to cover."

—Ty Bollinger, Founder of The Truth About Cancer

"Thank God for Dr. Leland Stillman! He has the courage to say out loud what many doctors have witnessed but dare not admit publicly. From the detrimental effects of aluminum in our vaccines to the fallout from the radiation we're exposed to, Stillman sheds light on what has led to our current autoimmunity epidemic. And, importantly, he offers us a lifeline for addressing it. This book is for anyone who is feeling stuck, sick, or hopeless."

—Hilda Labrada Gore, "Holistic Hilda," former host/producer of the *Wise Traditions* podcast

"Dr. Stillman has written a patient's guide that the pharmaceutical industry hopes you or your doctor never read."

—Dr. Patrick Lovegrove, author of *Healthy Aging for the Carolinas and Beyond*

"Dr. Stillman's book is a direct threat to what institutionalized medical care has to say about the human body and our ability and design to heal."

—ASHLEE ROWLAND, HOLISTIC NUTRITIONIST

"I am the Amy featured in this book. When I was first diagnosed with multiple sclerosis, I was overwhelmed and told there was no real path to recovery. I have since experienced firsthand what happens when you address the root causes of autoimmune disease. I wish I had a resource like this at the beginning of my healing journey. This book provides the direction I didn't have then."

—AMY ARP, MS, MEDICAL PHYSIOLOGY,
HEALTH COACH AT STILLMAN MD

THE END OF AUTOIMMUNITY

The End of Autoimmunity

Cutting-Edge Tactics for Energy, Vitality, and Longevity

Leland Stillman, MD

HOUNDSTOOTH PRESS

THE END OF AUTOIMMUNITY
Cutting-Edge Tactics for Energy, Vitality, and Longevity

FIRST EDITION

ISBN 978-1-5445-5251-4 *Hardcover*
978-1-5445-5250-7 *Paperback*
978-1-5445-5252-1 *Ebook*

This book is dedicated to my wife, Michelle, and my son, Benjamin. Every day with you is a joy. I love you both more than words can express.

Contents

A Note to the Reader

The information in this book reflects my clinical observations and the experiences of patients who have worked with me under medical supervision. It is educational in nature and is not intended as medical advice, nor as a substitute for the care of a qualified healthcare practitioner.

Nothing in this book is intended to diagnose, treat, cure, or prevent any disease. The FDA has not evaluated any statements herein.

The patient stories in this book represent real outcomes from real patients. They are not typical results. Individual results vary based on many factors, including the severity and duration of illness, adherence to the framework, and individual biochemistry.

I have a financial interest in some of the products and services I recommend. I disclose this where relevant throughout the text and online.

By reading this book, you acknowledge that you are responsible for your own health decisions and will consult qualified healthcare practitioners before implementing any protocol described here.

Introduction

WHAT THIS BOOK IS ABOUT

"The greatest medicine of all is teaching people how not to need it."

—Hippocrates

This book is about how we diagnose and treat autoimmune disease in our practice. Several years ago, when I started my own practice, I naturally attracted patients with autoimmunity. They were frustrated by their symptoms and looking for better answers than drugs and surgeries. They wanted root cause medicine. Our practice grew by word of mouth based on the results they saw.

Why autoimmunity? Autoimmune diseases steal the best years of many productive, driven, and conscientious people. They can't stand being tired, foggy, or inflamed. They can't stand the disfiguring skin rashes of psoriasis, vitiligo, or eczema. They can't stand the gut issues of Crohn's disease, ulcerative colitis, or lymphocytic colitis.

They want their lives back and many of them will go to great lengths to heal. This leads them to practices like ours, where we seek to do what other doctors call impossible—cure autoimmune diseases.

What makes our practice different? I have spent over twenty years studying natural and integrative medicine, and have been in practice for over twelve years. I have combined years of mentorship, study, and practice to create a single framework for treating autoimmune diseases. I have created a coherent system out of a collection of random protocols and practices.

I felt compelled to write this book by the exceptional results reported by patients thanks to our framework.

Between January and December of 2025, we surveyed every patient who completed a program or membership at our practice. A total of 103 patients responded (only a few did not). They reported an average improvement of 67 percent in general well-being. Specific domains showed even greater gains. Mood improved by 75 percent, stamina by 71 percent, cognition by 71 percent, digestion by 70 percent, energy by 70 percent, and sleep by 70 percent. These patients included children, the elderly, and adults of all ages who were single or married. We care for families with as many as ten children, and single individuals with no children. I believe our process can work for all kinds of people.

WHO THIS BOOK IS FOR

This book is for you if:

- You're exhausted, mentally "foggy," or dealing with gut issues, pain, or other symptoms that no one can fully explain.
- You have been diagnosed with an autoimmune condition or wonder if you have one.
- You would rather address the root causes of disease than

spend the rest of your life relying on drugs and surgeries to be able to function.

- You're the one in your family who researches health decisions for everyone else—often a mother or grandmother, sometimes homeschooling, or supporting a family business.
- You have already tried cleaning up your diet, fixing your sleep, and maybe even working with a clinician. You may have gone to every doctor in town and even started to travel to see doctors. Despite all your effort and hard work, you're still stuck far from where you want to be.
- You're skeptical of mainstream institutions and want a doctor who respects your faith, your conscience, and your freedom.
- You know there are no quick fixes or shortcuts to good health.

This book is not for everyone. It requires dedication. It asks you to change your diet, your environment, and your daily habits. It asks you to question what you've been told by institutions that may not have your best interests at heart. It asks you to take responsibility for your own health.

If you're looking for a magic pill or a thirty-day cure, this isn't it.

If you're ready to do the work, keep reading. In the pages ahead, I'll show you exactly what that work looks like, and why it's worth it for you and the people who depend on you.

A NOTE TO PRACTITIONERS

If you are a practitioner or coach of any kind, welcome. This book gives you the clinical framework we use. The companion resources at stillmanmd.com/autoimmunity include technical guides on everything in this book and more beyond it.

If you want to learn this system at a deeper level, look for the "For Practitioners" section in the companion resources.

WHAT YOU ACTUALLY WANT

Before we talk about diet, lifestyle, lab tests, or therapeutics, it helps to define what you're actually hoping will change.

I've learned from thousands of patient conversations that most of our patients want the same thing. They want to feel like themselves again. They want enough energy, mental clarity, and physical strength to be at their best for their friends, their family, and their calling.

Beyond this, they want three things.

First, they want a process that consistently delivers results. They don't want to waste time and money on things that don't work or that only offer fleeting improvement.

Second, they want results as quickly as possible, without sacrificing quality or durability. They're tired of being sick and tired, and they want to get back to living their lives as soon as possible.

Third, they want results that stand the test of time. They don't want to spend the rest of their life running in and out of doctors' offices, chasing one protocol after another.

They want a process that delivers what I call durable, significant results with the least amount of wasted effort and sacrifice.

That's the process I've been refining for over twenty years. That's what I've found patients want, and so that's what this book is about.

WHAT YOU'LL FIND HERE

This book shares our complete framework for addressing autoimmunity. It's the same framework we use daily in our practice.

You'll learn why autoimmunity has become an epidemic. You'll learn the principles that determine success or failure. You'll learn what's essential for a healthy immune system and the hazards that will ruin your immune system. You'll see how we diagnose and treat autoimmunity. You'll have a front-row seat to what we see in our practice every day.

Everything in this book is information I share with patients in our consults. I can't teach you everything I know, but I can show you the diet, lifestyle, testing, and treatment recommendations we use to get great results.

This is the manual for both patients and staff at our practice.

WHAT YOU WON'T FIND HERE

This book does not cover every supplement, medication, or therapy relevant to autoimmunity. I've focused on what delivers the best results in our practice.

There are many therapeutics that did not make it into this book. Chances are, it's not because I haven't heard of or tried them. I built our method from the ground up, starting with the most fundamental and progressing to the most advanced. I write about advanced therapeutics elsewhere. This book is where everyone should begin, because these are the things that matter most.

I built my practice and my reputation on one thing—results. I cannot afford for patients to not get well. Everything in this book has been tested in clinical practice with hundreds of real patients over many years. If you include the work of my mentors and predecessors, these tools and tactics have been tested over decades or even centuries of combined clinical experience.

You'll also notice I don't spend much time covering pharmaceutical drugs or surgical interventions. It's not because they never have value. This book focuses on the underlying factors that I believe drive autoimmunity in the first place. This is root cause medicine.

THE DIAGNOSIS DOESN'T MATTER AS MUCH AS YOU THINK

You might be wondering if this will help with your specific diagnosis. What if you don't even have a diagnosis yet?

The diagnosis matters less than you might think. Many of our patients come to us with nothing but a suspicion that something autoimmune is going on. We don't wait for a diagnosis to start working through the framework. Why would we? What matters is the process behind the diagnosis. I've found that our process works well across a wide range of diagnoses.

HOW TO USE THIS BOOK

This book is your guide to our process and framework. It is detailed enough to be helpful, brief enough to be practical, and impactful enough to be worth reading and taking action on. That being said, I have prepared many companion resources beyond this book that you may find useful.

You will find your companion resources at stillmanmd.com/autoimmunity.

The two most important are:

1. **The Repair Deficit Survey** to see where you stand right now
2. **The 14-Day Reset** to start building your foundation immediately

Start with those two. The rest of the companion resources you'll find there are supplementary to this book. Not everyone will need them, but many people will and so I took the time to write them.

You can also submit questions for our Q&A's at stillmanmd.com/autoimmunity. I can't promise I will answer every question, but I will do my best.

If you prefer to scan a QR code rather than type out the link address, here it is:

Take the Repair Deficit Survey now. Write down your score. We'll come back to it later.

WHY I WRITE

"I have come that they might have life, and have it more abundantly."

—John 10:10

My hope for you, as for my patients, is that you will have life and have it in abundance. I wrote this book when demand at our practice exceeded supply. Whole families fly across the country to see us, usually after starting with just one family member. No matter how much we grow the team, there are always more people to serve than we can accommodate.

I can't be everyone's doctor, but I can be your guide. The world you and I live in is changing quickly. We face new toxins, stresses, and threats to our bodies and freedoms every year. What I share here is what has held up over years of practice. As we learn more, I want to keep sharing my insights and experiences with you.

That's why this book always points you back to stillmanmd.com/autoimmunity. That's where I publish updates, answer your questions, and share new resources. If this book helps you, I hope you'll subscribe to my blog and newsletter so I can keep sharing my best information and insights with you.

Thank you for reading and supporting my work.

In gratitude,
Dr. Stillman

CHAPTER 1

How We View Autoimmunity

"To see things in the seed, that is genius."

—Lao Tzu

Until recently, autoimmunity was rare. We have to search the pages of medical history carefully to find any mention of it before modern times.[1]

What is autoimmunity? It's a disease process in which the immune system becomes confused and attacks the patient's cells, organs, and tissues.[2]

Why does this happen?

It can't be genetic.[3] Genes don't change in a few generations.[4]

You are probably old enough to appreciate how our immune systems have deteriorated in recent years.

Our grandparents grew up in a time when no one had allergies or autoimmune diseases. They had never heard of peanut allergies, autism, and many other modern childhood illnesses.[5]

Our parents grew up in a time when most kids were

healthy. Childhood diseases were on the rise, but most children needed little more than the occasional home remedy, let alone a prescription.

Today, our youth are dealing with a crisis of mental and physical disease. Much of this disease is autoimmune in nature.

The numbers tell the story. Today, over fifty million Americans have been diagnosed with at least one autoimmune disease. That's one in six people. In just one generation, blood markers of autoimmunity in the United States have risen from about one in nine people to approximately one in six—a 50 percent jump. If this pace continues for three more generations, these blood markers will be positive in one of every two Americans.[6]

This is not sustainable. We must put an end to the epidemic of autoimmunity, not just for ourselves, but for future generations.

What has changed in the last few generations to explain the explosive rise of autoimmunity?

Our diets, lifestyles, and environments have changed radically. These changes are driving the modern epidemic of autoimmunity.

As I studied the results from our practice and the scientific literature on autoimmunity, I became convinced that autoimmunity arises due to what we call "repair deficit." This is the difference between the damage we accumulate in our cells and tissues, and our ability to repair that damage. When damage exceeds repair capacity, a repair deficit appears.

What causes the damage that creates a repair deficit? I divided the root causes of autoimmunity into three categories: Metabolic Imbalances, Toxins and Stress, and Infections. This led me to create a three-step process for addressing these root causes: Nourish, Detoxify, Purify.

I needed a framework to turn this theory into practice. Our framework is Principles, Essentials, Hazards, Diagnostics, and Therapeutics.

Principles are what you believe about yourself, others, and our world. They are your values, your behavior, and your moral code.

Essentials are the things we must do to maintain good health. These are habits without which anyone will succumb to chronic disease.

Hazards are things that will destroy your health no matter what you do. They must be eliminated, mitigated, or minimized to achieve good health.

Diagnostics are how we test for the root causes of disease, as well as their manifestations. This includes lab testing, diagnostic imaging, vital signs, and more.

Therapeutics are how we treat disease. At our practice, this includes nutritional supplements, medications, and changes to diet, lifestyle, or environment.

If you don't understand what's behind autoimmunity, it's impossible to create a unified framework to address it. That's why it's important that you understand the concept of repair deficit.

If you don't understand what the root causes of autoimmunity are, you may miss one or more of them. This leads to what I call therapeutic failure—patients who do not get well.

When you have a theory as to why disease occurs (repair deficit and the root causes of disease), you can create a process (Nourish, Detoxify, Purify) and a framework (Principles, Essentials, Hazards, Diagnostics, Therapeutics) that turn theory into action.

We'll keep coming back to these ideas throughout the book.

To explain the concept, process, and framework, I'd like to

share a story of what's possible when you approach autoimmunity from this perspective.

ONE WOMAN WHO REVERSED THE INCURABLE

Amy Arp was headed for medical school when one day she woke up and could not feel her legs.

She was rushed to the hospital. The neurologist ordered an MRI. The scan showed lesions scattered throughout her brain and spinal cord. She was diagnosed with multiple sclerosis, an autoimmune disease that attacks the central nervous system.

The prognosis was grim. She would likely end up in a wheelchair. She wouldn't be able to care for children, if she could even have them. If she managed to complete medical school, her career would be short.

She was in her late twenties. She was devastated.

Why do I believe this happened to Amy?

Amy grew up in Salinas, California. Salinas is a farming town in the heart of California's agricultural belt. She was surrounded by pesticides from the day she was born.

She had severe allergies as a child. For years, she received allergy shots. Each shot may have contained aluminum as an adjuvant. The dose per shot is small, but over years of weekly injections, the cumulative aluminum burden can become extreme. This is in addition to the aluminum she received with her childhood vaccines. There are strong links between aluminum and multiple sclerosis.[7]

She went to college and studied biology. Like most college students, she drank sodas and other beverages out of aluminum cans. She ate processed food from dining halls and restaurants. Aluminum and other toxic chemicals are known to leach into our food from packaging materials.[8]

After college, she took two years to do mission work in El Salvador. She lived in conditions where parasitic infections are common. She likely picked up parasites there, though she didn't know it at the time.

She returned to the United States, got married, and started a job in corporate finance. Then she pursued her dream of becoming a doctor. She quit her job and applied to a master's program at Loyola University in Chicago.

That's when she lost sensation from her waist down. She found out she had been accepted to her top program while in the hospital being diagnosed. Her doctors told her she would soon be wheelchair-bound due to the location of the lesions in her brain and spinal cord.

How did Amy respond to her new diagnosis?

First, she cried for weeks.

Then, she refused to accept what doctors told her. She set out to make a complete recovery. She learned about environmental toxins. She learned about the role of nutrition in immune function. She learned about parasites and how infections may drive autoimmunity, particularly multiple sclerosis.

People thought she was crazy. She refused to listen to them. She found stories of others who had overcome multiple sclerosis, and she studied them intently. She learned everything she could.

She changed everything.

She cleaned up her diet. She eliminated processed foods, gluten, and dairy. She started eating organic, nutrient-dense whole foods prepared at home.

She removed sources of toxins from her life and implemented detoxification protocols.

She eliminated parasites from her time in El Salvador.

She focused relentlessly on giving her body what it needed

to repair itself. She devoted a year to the process. Her progress was not linear. She endured through good days and bad days.

Her symptoms resolved. Her follow-up MRIs showed resolution of active lesions. She never needed a wheelchair.

After her recovery, she completed her master's program and was headed to medical school with a 4.0 GPA. When she refused to take the COVID-19 vaccine, her physician mentors informed her that she would not be able to go to medical school. Based on her research, she had concluded the vaccine might cause her to relapse into multiple sclerosis. She was also concerned about the lack of long-term safety data.

Amy was deeply disappointed. She had worked for years to go to medical school. She held to her convictions and gave up her dream of becoming a doctor.

She looked for alternatives. She took a training program with me. I quickly recognized her potential and hired her to run our autoimmunity program.

Amy has been symptom-free for seven years as of this writing (2026). She recently had her first child. She now spends her days helping others who struggle with autoimmunity.

Amy and I recorded a two-part podcast about her journey. You can hear her story in her own words at stillmanmd.com/autoimmunity.

Amy's story is extreme, which is why I share it. It shows what's possible, even in severe cases. But you don't need lesions on an MRI to benefit from the information in this book. You don't need a formal diagnosis. If you're exhausted for reasons no one can explain, if your thinking feels slow, if you've gained weight you can't lose, if your mood has tanked, or you're struggling with bloating, abdominal pain, and other gut issues, then this book is for you. The root causes of autoimmunity are always the same.

THE ROOTS OF HER DISEASE

What were the root causes of Amy's multiple sclerosis? I view all diseases as arising from three root causes.

The first cause is metabolic imbalances. Metabolic imbalances include both nutrient deficiencies and excesses (both are important). Years of processed food and stress depleted the nutrients her body needed for repair. Her immune system was malnourished. The immune system must be properly nourished to function properly.

The second root cause is toxins and stress. She was exposed to pesticides from agriculture, aluminum from vaccines and allergy shots, and heavy metals from processed food, air pollution, and water pollution. These toxins accumulated in her tissues. Combine these with stresses like artificial light, sleep deprivation, and psychological stress (just to name a few), and the immune system can eventually lose control and start to attack your own cells and tissues. When enough toxins and stress have accumulated, the immune system can lose control and target our own cells and tissues.[9]

The third cause is infections. She eliminated parasites she presumably picked up in El Salvador as she took high doses of anti-parasitics. Parasites produce proteins that mimic human tissue. This is called molecular mimicry.[10] Her immune system had to distinguish between parasite and self. When the immune system is impaired by malnutrition, toxins, and stress, infections can take root. When the immune system attempts to eliminate infections, malnutrition, toxins, and stress can cause it to mistake host tissue for the infection, due to molecular mimicry. The result is autoimmunity.[11]

Most people think autoimmunity is the body attacking itself for no reason. This is only part of the story.

Imagine you're in outer space watching the surface of the

planet. Disaster strikes. Wildfires, hurricanes, volcanic eruptions, or a meteorite. You watch rescuers and aid convoys pour into the affected area. From space, how different does this look from a military operation or an attack?

What if autoimmunity is your body's best attempt to rescue damaged cells and tissues?

I believe that autoimmunity is your body's attempt to repair damaged tissues and resolve chronic inflammation. Your immune system is confused, but it's responding to real threats like toxins and infections. It's doing so while malnourished and stressed out. It should be no surprise that under these circumstances, it can make mistakes.

The problem isn't that your immune system is broken. The problem is that the damage exceeds your capacity to repair it.

This is what I call a repair deficit.

REPAIR DEFICIT: THE CORE CONCEPT

We view autoimmunity as the result of what we call "repair deficit." I learned this concept from one of my mentors, Dr. Russell Jaffe, a pioneer and champion of integrative medicine.

What is a repair deficit? It's when damage to the body is accumulating faster than your body can repair it.

Think of your health like a bank account. Every stress is a withdrawal, whether it's a late night, a processed meal, or a season of pushing through when your body is begging you to rest.

Some withdrawals are small. You barely notice them. Others are dramatic enough to wreck your credit and wipe out your savings. Sometimes we think we just need a twenty-dollar tire patch when we actually need a $20,000 rebuild. The worst thing to do in that situation is to try to get away with the twenty-dollar tire patch—this just leads to more suffering and expense in the long run.

Your body can recover from these withdrawals, but it needs deposits—nutrients, rest, sunlight, clean water, time to heal. The problem is that deposits are slow and withdrawals are fast. One sleepless night can take days to recover from. One stressful season can take months. And the older we get, the slower the deposits accumulate.

Every day in our practice, I see people in the prime of life whose accounts are exhausted. Their spouses, children, and parents are counting on them. Their colleagues, bosses, and employees rely on them. Their purpose is out there, calling to them.

Meanwhile, they've run out of energy, positivity, patience, brain power, and physical strength. They try to make another withdrawal, only to find out their wallet is empty and their cards are maxed out.

The bad news is that you might have a significant repair deficit to pay off.

The good news is that now you know what the problem is, and you can solve it.

Anything that injures the body or delays repair creates a repair deficit. If you rest, recover, and nourish your body afterward, your body can fully repair itself. This book will show you how.

If you make a habit of depriving yourself of sleep, nourishing food, a clean environment, and time to rest and regenerate, then your repair deficit grows.

Repair deficit gives rise to chronic inflammation. As damage accumulates, the body responds by creating inflammation. The purpose of inflammation is to trigger repair. When resources for repair are inadequate, inflammation becomes chronic.[12]

Chronic inflammation is a hallmark of autoimmune conditions.[13]

When the repair deficit is extreme enough for long enough, the safety mechanisms of the immune system can fail. The immune system may react against your cells and tissues. But this reaction is an attempt to repair damaged cells and tissues, not a random malfunction.

In our practice, we work with patients to address the root causes of disease that create a repair deficit. This is our process—Nourish, Detoxify, Purify.

THE PROCESS: NOURISH, DETOXIFY, PURIFY

If you ask Amy what she did during the time when her symptoms resolved, she will give you a long list. All of these things fall into three categories.

She optimized nutrition to support her immune and nervous systems.

She reduced her toxic burden.

She eliminated parasites that she presumably picked up in El Salvador.

Amy Nourished, Detoxified, and Purified her body for an entire year. Her MRI now shows a perfectly healthy brain and spinal cord. Today, seven years later, she has no signs or symptoms of multiple sclerosis.

Her doctors called it "luck." They presented to her at the outset, with certainty, that she would lead a short life of progressive disability.

I find the idea that Amy's recovery was "luck" to be ridiculous.

If you want to know how Amy beat multiple sclerosis, listen to our two-part podcast on her journey at stillmanmd.com/autoimmunity.

THE FRAMEWORK: TURNING THEORY INTO PRACTICE

Amy was in her twenties when her health collapsed. You might be in your forties or fifties, juggling your health while caring for kids, aging parents, or both, and carrying the quiet weight of being the one everyone turns to when something is wrong. You might be in your sixties, seventies, or even eighties, caring for a spouse, while watching out for children, grandchildren, and great-grandchildren. The details are different. The pattern is the same.

The three root causes of disease are the same in each case. They combine to create a repair deficit. The root causes of disease give rise to our process—Nourish, Detoxify, Purify. This is the process we use to resolve a repair deficit.

I created a framework to hand to patients as they go through this process. The framework makes this workable in daily life. I organized the rest of this book into five parts to explain this framework, which consists of Principles, Essentials, Hazards, Diagnostics, and Therapeutics.

Principles (Chapter 2) are the ways of thinking and behaving that make this work.

Essentials (Chapter 3) are the daily choices you make to optimize your health and your immune system.

Hazards (Chapter 4) are the toxins and stresses of life that undermine your health and your immune system.

Diagnostics (Chapter 5) are the tests and surveys that guide our choices.

Therapeutics (Chapter 6) are the specific tools we use to move patients forward, from illness to wellness.

The best analogy for this is that of repairing a home that's been damaged. The concept is that maintenance was deferred for too long (repair deficit). The process is to bring in building materials, remove damaged or compromised building materials, and then install the new materials. The framework is like the blueprint or plan for the whole project.

In the next chapter, I will show you exactly how patients use this process and framework to achieve their goals.

YOUR NEXT STEP

Before moving to Chapter 2, take the Repair Deficit Survey at stillmanmd.com/autoimmunity, if you haven't already.

It takes two minutes and will give you a baseline to track how your repair deficit changes as you work through this framework.

Now, let's look at the three principles that determine whether patients get great results.

CHAPTER 2

Principles

"Strategy without tactics is the slowest road to victory. Tactics without strategy is the noise before defeat."

—Sun Tzu, *The Art of War*

There are three principles that I believe matter most when it comes to healing from autoimmunity.

They are:

- Commit to a Framework
- Climb the Therapeutic Tree
- Keep Doing What Works

When I first set out to create a single framework for treating autoimmunity, I did not think much of principles. But the more I considered the most remarkable case studies from our practice, the more I realized that these were deeply principled people. Their success was not a matter of chance. It was not a matter of just going through the motions. I believe their success was rooted in their principles.

What are principles? They are how we live our lives. They are what we believe about ourselves and our world. They are how we speak, think, behave, and treat ourselves and others.

Patients and practitioners are attracted to what I call "tactics." Tactics like "take magnesium for sleep," or "eat fiber for gut health." Strategy is how you approach healing altogether. Do you stay positive when things get tough? Do you quit at the first hint of failure? These are principles. I think of principles as being akin to strategy, while treatments are akin to tactics.

I think healing starts with principles—with strategy.

There are many principles that I believe matter to the practice of medicine. Maybe one day I'll write a book about all of them. For our purposes, there are three that I think are most important.

As I considered these principles, I realized that they grew out of our deepest desires as patients (and practitioners).

What patients want most is great results—that much is obvious.

But they want more than just great results.

Patients want great results, consistently. The lower the likelihood of success, the less interested they become. They don't want to waste time, money, and energy on protocols and procedures that don't work consistently. They all know that nothing is certain, but the more consistent the results, the more valuable the process or procedure will be to them.

Patients want great results quickly. All we have, in the end, is time. Patients want to get well as quickly as possible, without compromising the quality of their results.

Patients want great results that last. After all the time, effort, and sacrifice that goes into getting well, patients want results that stand the test of time. There is little more discouraging or disheartening than, "going backwards"—watching hard-won gains evaporate, often for no apparent reason.

The three principles I chose to include in this book are the ones that I have found maximize the likelihood of success (consistent results), increase the speed at which results are achieved (fast results), and that yield results that stand the test of time (results that last).

If you're going to get great results consistently, then you need to Commit to a Framework.

If you're going to get great results quickly, then you need to Climb the Therapeutic Tree.

If you're going to get great results that last, then you need to Keep Doing What Works.

There are three specific patients who came to mind as I thought through these principles. I will share their stories with you in this chapter as examples of what it means to embody these principles.

A NOTE ON HOW TO READ THIS CHAPTER

This chapter teaches three principles through real patient stories. I've streamlined the case studies here to keep you focused on what matters most.

For those who want the complete picture with every lab value and protocol detail, I've included expanded case studies in the companion resources at stillmanmd.com/autoimmunity. Here, I'll show you the results, explain what we did, and teach you the principles.

HOW TO GET GREAT RESULTS CONSISTENTLY

If you're going to get great results consistently, then you need to Commit to a Framework. I believe great results are most likely when patients are committed to a single therapeutic framework. Repair deficit is a concept—a unifying theme of why autoimmunity occurs. Nourish, Detoxify, and Purify is a process—how we get from illness to wellness. Our framework (Principles, Essentials, Hazards, Diagnostics, Therapeutics) guides us through that process.

I often see patients picking and choosing their therapeutics from different frameworks. They take this doctor's supplement, another doctor's detox protocol, and a third doctor's in-office procedure (think surgeries, stem cells, and more). This often ends in disappointment and frustration. Why do I caution you against this approach?

Imagine you are coaching a professional sports team. Your general manager hires additional coaches, who give your players instructions that conflict with yours. It isn't that they aren't good coaches—it's that at the end of the day, you need one coach. A football team needs one quarterback, a soccer team needs one goalie, and an army needs one general. Sometimes two is worse than one.

Every great physician I know has a system. It might just be in their head. Rarely is it available in a book or a series of blog posts. But they turn it over in their mind all day. It makes sense to them. It is what they base their reputation and their practice on.

The trouble with mixing and matching frameworks (having two coaches) is you wind up with duplicate therapies, conflicting therapies, and sometimes "too much" for the body to handle. I see many, many patients hop from framework to framework, implementing parts of each. Their results are lackluster. Sometimes I liken it to baking a cake. Imagine if you skipped ingredients and mixed and matched recipes. Would you expect the cake to turn out well?

I have observed that people who do not commit to a single

framework often skip critical elements of the framework. Imagine a team that works only on technique. They might have the prettiest passes and shots in the game, but a team that balances technique with physical conditioning will run them into the ground. Imagine a team that only focuses on physical conditioning and over-trains. They will fail on game day against a team that practiced less, rested more, and had a better technique.

Coach John Wooden is arguably the most successful coach in the history of sports. Wooden created what he called his "pyramid of success." The pyramid consisted of blocks and mortar that were key character traits or virtues, like honesty, friendship, and poise. He worked on this framework for his whole career. He had a script for every practice. His team did not practice as much as many teams, as he believed shorter, more intense practices were more productive. Yet he had an unmatched record of success. He won ten national championships in twelve years, including seven in a row between 1967 and 1973. During his tenure, his team had an eighty-eight-game winning streak, four perfect seasons, and thirty-eight straight tournament wins.

The word "doctor" means "teacher." The word "coach" originally referred to someone who "carried" a student through a course of study or exam. I believe we should help you achieve success as your coaches and teachers. We are not mechanics. You are not cars or robots. We cannot just give you "orders" and expect you to win. Coach Wooden was a man who developed players. And he and his players did what others would have called "impossible." Wooden credited their success to specific virtues, many of which are necessary to Commit to a Framework of any kind.

"The patient must combat the disease along with the physician."

—Hippocrates

Every great testimonial or story from our practice came from a patient who committed to the framework. They did the boring, tedious parts of the framework (like taking walks, resting, and preparing healthy food) just as intently as they did the exciting parts (high doses of nutrients, pharmaceuticals, or hormones).

There are many practitioners who do not have a framework, or are early in the process of developing one. Working with them feels like throwing spaghetti at the wall. You may feel like there is no rhyme or reason to their method. You may feel like, after their first few recommendations or appointments, there is nothing more to do. Every practitioner has depth to their framework. Some frameworks are more robust and better developed than others. Regardless of which framework you pick, commit to it.

Complex cases require frameworks. Let me show you what committing to a framework looks like.

JOHN'S STORY: COMMITTING TO THE FRAMEWORK

John came to see me in 2022. His son, a fellow physician, referred him to me. John was a former executive who, rather than retiring to play golf and travel, had become a college professor. He loved teaching. He cared deeply about people. He was the kind of man anyone would have wanted as a father or grandfather. He was kind, thoughtful, determined, and principled. His family wanted to see him restored to good health.

John was over six feet and weighed just 150 pounds. He was losing weight. He had suffered from gastric ulcers for years, culminating in a partial gastrectomy. Part of his stomach had been removed. He could barely eat. He could barely digest what he did eat due to acid-blocking medications. He was constipated, which made eating even more painful.

Multiple systems were failing. He was anemic. His hormones were at rock bottom. He was wasting away.

Here's what his baseline labs showed:

- Hemoglobin was 9.4 g/dL. Normal is 13.2 to 17.1 g/dL. This is a severe case of anemia.
- His white blood cell count was 3.2 k/uL. Normal is 3.8–10.8.
- Free T3 was 2.1 pg/mL. Optimal is over 3.4 pg/mL. He had low thyroid function.
- Testosterone was 335 ng/dL. Optimal is 800 to 1400 ng/dL. His testosterone was half of what it should have been.
- DHEA-S was 14 mcg/dL. Optimal is 400 to 600 mcg/dL. His adrenals were exhausted.
- His stool testing revealed poor enzyme production, poor fat absorption, inflammation, dysbiosis, and *Yersinia enterocolitica*—a pathogenic bacteria.
- His urine showed B-6 deficiency.
- His blood showed deficiencies in proline, copper, magnesium, potassium, and zinc.

John committed to the framework. He was consistent in the daily habits and actions I recommended to him. He showed up to every appointment ready to report on what he had done since our last appointment, and ready for new instructions on what to do next. He was one of the most dedicated and focused patients I have ever worked with.

He nourished his body. He changed his diet completely. He needed carbohydrates for muscle gain, not the low-carb diet he'd been following. He added oats, nuts, seeds, root vegetables, cooked greens, and bone broths. He started targeted supplementation with B-6, magnesium, zinc, and collagen peptides.

He detoxified his body. He weaned off his acid-blocking

medications. He eliminated allergic triggers in his diet based on blood testing.

He purified his body. We treated the pathogenic bacteria with antibiotics followed by microbiome restoration. He added enzymes, bile acids, and herbs to heal his gut lining.

He also added red and infrared light therapy and spent more time in the sunlight.

Four months later, the results were incredible.

- His hemoglobin rose from 9.4 to 13.0 g/dL—approaching the normal range.
- His white blood cell count rose to 3.9 k/uL—within the normal range.
- His magnesium, potassium, proline, and organic acids all improved.
- He started gaining muscle.
- He restored healthy, daily bowel movements.
- He could eat again, without discomfort.

His hemoglobin continued to rise, eventually reaching 14.6 g/dL. A thirty-year anemia resolved in less than a year while he was a patient at our practice.

John came more and more alive every time I spoke to him.

Why did this work when nothing else had for thirty years?

John committed to the framework. He nourished his body with proper food and targeted supplements. He detoxified by fixing his diet and removing medications that blocked digestion. He purified by clearing the pathogenic bacteria.

John's commitment and consistency led to some of the most incredible results I have ever seen in practice. He did everything I recommended, exactly as I recommended it. He did not skip steps or procrastinate.

John's complete case study—iron panels, organic acids, mineral status, and exact supplement protocols—can be found in the Chapter 2 companion resources at stillmanmd.com/autoimmunity.

SELF-ASSESSMENT: ARE YOU COMMITTED TO A FRAMEWORK?

Answer the following questions. Pay attention to how you feel as you read them, and how you feel about your answers.

Are you struggling to do the hard work that's needed to be healthy? Yes / No / Sometimes

Have you worked with multiple practitioners, but never fully trusted one of them? Yes / No

Have you dabbled in more than one framework at a time and been disappointed in the results? Yes / No

Have you gotten temporary improvements that eventually faded away? Yes / No

Do you feel like you run from tire patch to tire patch, or crutch to crutch, wearing one out after another? Yes / No

What feelings come up as you answer these questions? How do you feel about your answers?

If you answered "yes" or "sometimes" to three or more questions above, commit to this framework for three to six months and track your progress every two weeks using the Repair Deficit Survey.

Patients who commit to our framework with enough intensity over a long enough period of time turn into our best testimonials and case studies. This is not a guarantee. Individual results vary. That does not change the fact that committing to a framework and following through on its implementation is a common feature among the most successful patients.

If you don't find answers to your questions about our framework here, look for them in the companion resources at stillmanmd.com/autoimmunity.

HOW TO GET GREAT RESULTS FASTER

Once you have a framework, you have to move through it. You have to start at the beginning, build a foundation, and then work your way to the end.

In our practice, we call this, "Climbing the Therapeutic Tree."

I think of therapeutics as being on a "tree." At the top of the tree are expensive, impractical, difficult, and even dangerous treatments. At the bottom of the tree are simple, cheap, easy, obvious, and even free treatments. For example, we have had patients travel all over the world (Japan, Austria, and Germany most notably) for treatments like stem cells or plasmapheresis. These treatments are at the top of the therapeutic tree. You could run comprehensive labs and receive a personalized supplement protocol based on your results (this is our standard practice). This would be the middle of the therapeutic tree. We also encourage our patients to pick the low-hanging fruit on the therapeutic tree, like taking walks, getting plenty of sleep, taking time for relaxation and positive social connection, and eating whole, highly nutritious food.

Many patients start at the top of the therapeutic tree. We sometimes call these therapeutics "shiny objects." If a therapeutic has a paid advertisement of any kind, it is a shiny object. There is nothing wrong with shiny objects, but too many people make their wellness about shiny objects while neglecting low-hanging fruit.

Some patients develop what we call "shiny object syndrome." I view this as a symptom of a larger problem. Their health is failing, and they are grasping at anything that offers them hope. But if your house is falling apart, you have to take a long, sober, and hard look at the foundation, the roof, the walls, the plumbing, or the electrical wiring. Usually, that is where the problem is. A shiny object might keep the wind and rain out for a night or two, but it won't fix a broken foundation.

We naturally gravitate toward shiny objects. This isn't a character flaw, it's just part of our nature. There's nothing wrong with climbing to the top of the therapeutic tree—in fact, it's arguably the best thing to do. But what we have observed time and again is that patients who skip the middle and low branches of the tree get the worst and most fleeting results. Patients who start at the bottom and work their way up get the best results.

Our framework guides patients up the therapeutic tree starting at the bottom and culminating at the top. You'll find my articles and thoughts on advanced therapeutics at stillmanmd.com/autoimmunity. If it's worth flying across the country or the world for, I'll take the time to write about it. If you have specific questions, feel free to submit them for a Q&A.

Here is what Climbing the Therapeutic Tree looks like in practice.

MEREDITH'S STORY: CLIMBING THE THERAPEUTIC TREE

Meredith Oke came to see me in 2020, struggling with severe fatigue. She was in her prime but felt like life was passing her by. Her husband worked globally, and their family had lived in Hong Kong, France, and Canada. During their travels, she had searched desperately for answers about why she was exhausted.

While trying to figure out how to restore her energy, she had to raise three children and make the most of her time with her husband when he wasn't traveling for work.

She immersed herself in the scientific literature on health and light. She tried light therapy. She bought blue blockers to help her sleep. She stopped wearing sunglasses and got more sunlight.

She saw about a 50 percent improvement. Then her progress stalled.

This is what I call therapeutic failure. The interventions that got her to 50 percent couldn't get her any further. This is when you need to climb higher on the therapeutic tree.

When Meredith came to me, she had already picked the low-hanging fruit. She was ready for the next level.

We started with breathing mechanics. Within days of fixing her dysfunctional breathing mechanics, her energy and mental clarity improved.

Her labs revealed multiple abnormalities linked to fatigue:

- Homogentisic acid was 9 mmol/mol creatinine. The ideal is below 8.0. This indicated a vitamin C deficiency.
- Kynurenic acid was 8.6 mmol/mol creatinine. Ideal is below 6.0. This indicated B-6 deficiency.
- Omega-3 index was 5.8 percent. Optimal is above 8.0 percent. This indicated omega-3 deficiency.
- Methylmalonic acid was 1.1 mmol/mol creatinine. Ideal is below 1.0. This indicated borderline B-12 deficiency.
- Lipid peroxides were 7.5 micromol/g creatinine. Ideal is below 6.0. This indicated excess free radical production and a deficiency of antioxidant defenses.
- Zinc was 98.7 mcg/dL. Ideal is above 105. This indicated a borderline zinc deficiency.

- Krebs cycle metabolites were borderline elevated. This indicated a sluggish metabolism.
- Her amino acids were depleted across the board, particularly proline, glycine, serine, asparagine, glutamine, arginine, and threonine.

Her body did not have what it needed to resolve a repair deficit.

She nourished herself with targeted supplements, specifically vitamin C, B-6, fish oil, selenium, and amino acids.

She addressed her environment. She found mold in her house and immediately remediated it.

She changed her diet. She had been eating foods that triggered inflammation. We eliminated them.

She added red light therapy panels, an infrared sauna, and light therapy patches.

She had her mercury amalgams removed.

If you're wondering what these things are, how they work, or if they are right for you, just relax. We will cover them all in due time. If you need more information than I provide in this book, just refer to the companion resources online. There, I intend to provide everything anyone could need in their journey with autoimmunity.

She added things gradually. She climbed the therapeutic tree quickly, not instantly. She understood the practical importance of laying a foundation. Too many patients go straight to the top and are underwhelmed or downright disappointed by a lack of durable, significant results.

Patience is one of the virtues we must cultivate to achieve anything worthwhile. Good health is no different. Your body cannot adapt to therapeutics instantly. Imagine you are baking a cake. Can you bake it at 500 degrees Fahrenheit and get the same results you would get at 350? Of course not. It might be crispy on the outside and gooey on the inside.

"Healing is a matter of time, but it is sometimes also a matter of opportunity."

—Hippocrates

Patients who get the best and fastest results start with the low-hanging fruit, and gradually ascend the tree at a speed they can sustain. They do not skip steps. They do not rush things.

Meredith didn't just take supplements. She didn't just start light therapy. She didn't just change her diet. She didn't just remediate mold. She did all of these things and more. She did them thoroughly, and she did them in order.

Six months after we started, she had regained the energy of her youth. Her labs had normalized. She felt so good that she started a practitioner training program.

Why did Meredith succeed?

She climbed the therapeutic tree, starting at the bottom and working her way up. She didn't try to do everything at once. She didn't rush to the top. She didn't start new habits or therapeutics only to abandon them the following week. She implemented what she could handle, as fast as she could, and then climbed higher up the therapeutic tree. This is how patients get better results faster.

Meredith recorded a three-part podcast with me about her journey. In part one, we cover her diagnosis and early years with her illness. In part two, we cover her journey as a patient at our practice. In part three, we cover her experience with light therapy and her favorite light therapy tools as a mother, wife, entrepreneur, and teacher.

You can hear Meredith's story in the Chapter 2 companion

resources at stillmanmd.com/autoimmunity. You'll also find her complete case study there, with exact lab details, supplement protocols, and more.

SELF-ASSESSMENT: WHERE ARE YOU ON THE THERAPEUTIC TREE?

Answer the following questions to find out where you are on the therapeutic tree. Pay attention to how you feel as you read each question, and how you feel about your answers.

Are there things you know you should do for your health that you aren't doing? Yes / No / Sometimes

Are you quick to take supplements or medications, but slow to change your habits and behaviors? Yes / No / Sometimes

Do you feel like your progress has stalled? Yes / No / Sometimes

Do you feel overwhelmed by everything you could do, but feel like you don't have clarity on what matters most? Yes / No / Sometimes

Do you spend a lot of time learning about health, but feel like no matter how much you learn, you are still stuck? Yes / No / Sometimes

What feelings come up as you answer these questions? How do you feel about your answers?

If you answered "yes" or "sometimes" to three or more questions here, commit to the 14-Day Reset and Daily Essentials Log. You will climb the tree, but start with the low-hanging fruit.

Meredith made it 50 percent of the way to her goal without medical help or supervision. She figured it out by doing her own research and picking the low-hanging fruit. This is what we will focus on in Chapters 3 and 4.

Most of our patients come to us already familiar with many of the low-hanging fruit of the therapeutic tree. They are gazing up at the tree, wondering how high they will have to climb and what it will cost them. They wonder if they can even reach the branches where their healing will occur.

Great practitioners guide their patients up the therapeutic tree with empathy and understanding, helping them achieve the best results possible, as fast as possible. This means not only helping them climb higher, but also helping them determine how high to climb, or when to come back down. You don't have to get to the top. You just have to achieve your goals. Great practitioners distinguish themselves not by heroic efforts and vast expense on the part of their patients, but by helping patients to get well as efficiently and completely as possible.

If you want to know what I tell our patients about any therapeutic, you'll either find it in this book or in the companion resources at stillmanmd.com/autoimmunity. If you don't find what you're looking for, submit a question for one of our Q&A's.

Once you have achieved your goals by climbing the therapeutic tree, you must consider how to maintain the progress you have made, or how to get great results that last.

HOW TO GET GREAT RESULTS THAT LAST

The secret to getting great results that last is to Keep Doing What Works. One of the trends we observe in the practice is that as patients recover their health, they tend to go back to old habits. The occasional glass of wine turns into the weekly glass of wine, and then twice weekly, and then a bottle every week. The occasional late-night out becomes a habit. Junk food creeps back in.

Our patients who get great results that last don't just adopt habits, supplements, or lifestyle changes for a season. They adopt a new diet and lifestyle for the rest of their life.

I am not saying that you cannot ever have a glass of wine, a late night out, or a "cheat meal." Every patient has a different tolerance for bad habits.

> *"Illnesses do not come upon us out of the blue. They are the consequence of small deadly sins against nature. When enough sins have accumulated, illnesses will suddenly appear."*
>
> —Hippocrates

When symptoms return, patients wonder, *What happened?* They may feel disappointed or disillusioned. A framework is only as strong as its execution over a long enough period of time. How many great sports teams win a championship, only to fall short the next season? How many great comeback stories are about getting back to doing what works?

Patients often want to quit their journey. The work doesn't feel worth it. They don't see major improvements with their daily walks, their healthy diet, or their careful sleep routine—all examples of low-hanging fruit. They feel like they are wasting their time. Or they recover their health and slip back into old habits, only to see their results fade away.

Great results take time. They require dedication. And they last for as long as that dedication does.

Here is a story about how to get great results that last.

EMILY'S STORY: KEEP DOING WHAT WORKS

Emily was thirty-two years old when she contacted me in December 2022. She had myasthenia gravis, an autoimmune disease where the immune system attacks the connections between nerves and muscles. Patients with myasthenia gravis gradually lose the strength to keep their eyes open, eat, swallow, and even breathe. Emily had a severe case and had already failed every drug available for myasthenia, plus the only surgery known to be effective for it. She experienced severe flares of her myasthenia shortly after receiving the first dose of one of the COVID-19 vaccines. Having run out of conventional options, she turned elsewhere for answers. She took Meredith Oke's training program, where I am still a member of the faculty, and shortly thereafter became a patient.

She was already doing everything right when she came to me. I had fewer suggestions for Emily than for almost any patient I have ever seen. She had a healthy diet. She had a healthy lifestyle.

We tested and found the root causes. Her urine showed B-6 and carnitine deficiencies. Her blood showed low magnesium, potassium, and zinc. We started a personalized supplement protocol.

Soon after starting personalized supplement protocols, Emily developed flu-like symptoms and skin rashes. We suspected these were detoxification reactions and that her body was starting to eliminate toxins, including heavy metals.

We repeated her hair test a few months later. The results were shocking.

Her aluminum had increased twenty-one-fold. Her mercury had tripled. Her copper had increased over threefold.

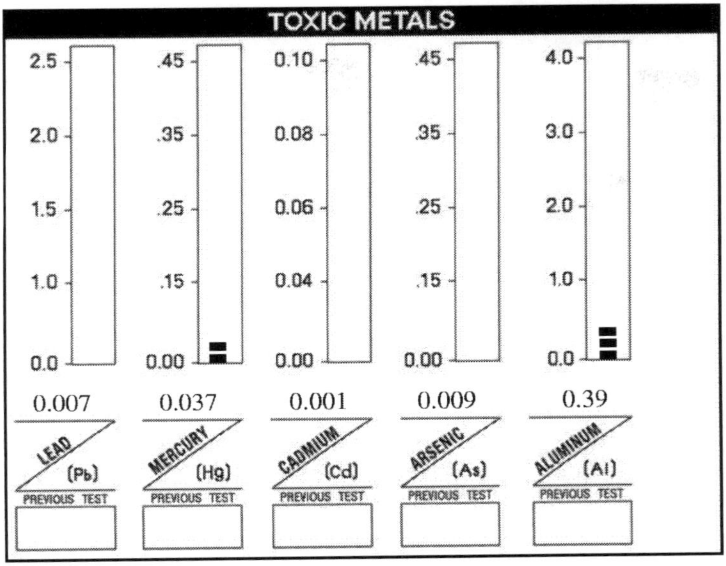

Figure 1. Initial Hair Metals

Her first hair test showed low heavy metal levels. You might expect this to mean that she had few, if any, heavy metals in her body.

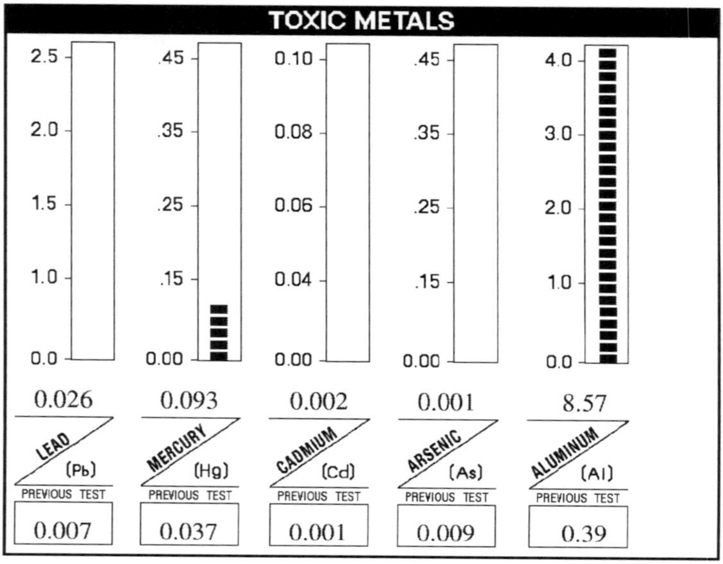

Figure 2. Follow Up Hair Metals

What could explain this sudden rise in heavy metals? Her body had been "hiding" her metals. When the body does not have the energy, due to nutritional deficiencies, toxic burden, or infection, heavy metal levels in the hair actually fall. As we Nourish, Detoxify, and Purify the body, heavy metal levels rise. If you're curious to learn more about this, check the companion resources for more information.

This is why from her first test to her second test, her heavy metal levels skyrocketed.

Most impressive of all was her aluminum elimination.[14]

Her first hair test showed an aluminum level of 390 mcg%.

Her second test showed a level of 8,570 mcg%.

Six months after her second test, her hair aluminum was 2,360 mcg%.

Her aluminum levels increased twenty-one-fold, or 2,197

percent, between her first and second test. Her mercury levels nearly tripled, and her lead levels nearly quadrupled.

The clinical results were life-changing. Over eighteen months, Emily went from unable to conceive, fatigued, and struggling with the symptoms of myasthenia gravis to symptom-free and pregnant. She gave birth to her first child the following summer. Her last myasthenia flare was before her massive metal elimination. She has been symptom-free for over two years (as of this writing) without drugs.

Why did Emily's results last?

She never went back to what made her sick in the first place. She committed to consistent daily action for eighteen months. She didn't quit when she had uncomfortable detox reactions. She trusted the process even when progress felt slow. She eliminated massive amounts of aluminum, copper, and mercury from her body. Her results have stood the test of time because she has not gone back to her old way of life.

Emily recorded a podcast with me about her journey. You'll find her full case study, including heavy metal and mineral eliminations, and her podcast at stillmanmd.com/autoimmunity.

SELF-ASSESSMENT: WILL YOUR RESULTS LAST?

Answer the following questions to see if your results will last. Pay attention to how you feel as you read each question, and how you feel about your answers.

Have you stopped doing things that were working because you reached your goals? Yes / No / Sometimes

Do you tend to ease up on healthy habits as soon as you feel a little better? Yes / No / Sometimes

Have you gone back to habits, environments, or lifestyle choices that made you sick in the first place? Yes / No / Sometimes

Do you feel like you only ever see brief improvements, rather than lasting results? Yes / No / Sometimes

What feelings come up as you answer these questions? How do you feel about your answers?

If you answered "yes" or "sometimes" to two or more of the above questions, commit to the 14-Day Reset and Daily Essentials Log, and take the Repair Deficit Survey every two weeks for three to six months. The work that got you better is the work that will keep you better.

The secret to great results that last might be best summed up in a simple phrase—fall in love with the process. Patients who get great results that last don't think about "having" to do this or that to maintain their wellness. They do it because they fall in love with it. If you've struggled to fall in love with what it takes to be healthy, then I encourage you to study our companion resources. I know how hard it can be to stick to new habits and choices, so I have done my best to come up with solutions that our patients can fall in love with. You'll find them all at stillmanmd.com/autoimmunity.

WHY THESE THREE PRINCIPLES MATTER

I reviewed dozens of cases from our practice in preparing this book. I see hundreds of patients each year, and I spend hours with each of them. Our most successful cases follow the three principles I've shared with you here. I could have written about dozens of other principles that I think matter, but these emerged in my mind as undoubtedly the three most important.

John, Meredith, and Emily achieved exceptional outcomes. By no means does following these principles guarantee success. I have seen many patients work as diligently as John, Meredith, or Emily, and see no benefit at all. But as Coach Wooden said, "The harder you work, the more luck you will have."

COMPANION RESOURCES FOR CHAPTER 2

If you're curious to learn more about John, Meredith, or Emily's cases, I encourage you to read their full case studies, available in the companion resources online.

I have also included additional case studies that may interest you, particularly if you have a diagnosis or symptom that John, Meredith, and Emily did not have. I have many more inspiring stories from our practice than I could include here.

You will find them all in the Chapter 2 companion resources at stillmanmd.com/autoimmunity.

WHAT COMES NEXT

Now that we have covered strategy, we can move on to tactics.

Chapter 3 covers what we call Essentials. These are the daily habits and choices that create good health and optimal immunity.

Chapter 4 covers what we call Hazards. These are things that undermine our health and directly cause autoimmunity.

Chapter 5 covers Diagnostics. These are the tests and tools we rely on in our practice to direct our efforts.

Chapter 6 covers Therapeutics. These are the supplements, medications, and procedures that we rely on to treat our patients with autoimmunity.

If you want to learn more about anything you read here, check the companion resources at stillmanmd.com/autoimmunity. If you don't find what you're looking for, you can submit your questions there as well.

YOUR NEXT STEP

You now understand the three principles that are key to getting great results consistently, quickly, and that last:

- Commit to a Framework
- Climb the Therapeutic Tree
- Keep Doing What Works

Before moving to Chapter 3, ask yourself honestly which principle you're most likely to violate. Cherry-picking parts of the framework? Skipping foundations or refusing to climb higher? Backsliding when you start feeling better?

Write it down. Keep it visible as you work through the rest of this book.

Then turn to Chapter 3 and begin with the Essentials.

CHAPTER 3

Essentials

"Patients should have rest, food, fresh air, and exercise—the quadrangle of health."

—Sir William Osler, MD

The essentials are essential. Without the essentials, people fall apart.

The patients who see the greatest improvements in our practice commit to the essentials first. They are like a foundation. Without them, you should expect results to shift, change, and even disappear. You might feel like you are chasing results that slip through your fingers as soon as you tighten your grasp.

This is why, after principles, we start with the essentials. I break them down into breathing, hydration, light, food, and exercise. There are many, many more essentials than these five topics, and each of these topics has subtopics that deserve more detailed explanation. This is why there are companion resources at stillmanmd.com/autoimmunity. Here, I cover the essentials I have found to have the greatest impact on patients at our practice.

GOOD, BETTER, BEST

Throughout this book, I will frame my approach in terms of Good, Better, and Best. Each of us has limited resources to spend in this life. These resources can fluctuate with the seasons of life. Above all, do not be discouraged if you cannot achieve *Best* right now. *Good* may be enough to achieve every hope and dream that you have. *Better* might not be practical for you. *Best* might be a wild dream. I encourage you to always seek to improve your circumstances, but in the meantime, "do what you can, where you are, with what you have," as President Teddy Roosevelt once said.

What do Good, Better, and Best look like when it comes to the essentials?

- Good means practicing what I call the 14-Day Reset.
- Better means digging deeper into the essentials outlined in this book and within the companion resources online.
- Best means optimizing your essentials with one-to-one medical guidance or expert coaching.

First, let me share with you the 14-Day Reset.

DR. STILLMAN'S 14-DAY RESET

I created the 14-Day Reset as a simple starting point for our patients.

It's easy for people to get overwhelmed on this journey. I have spent twenty years figuring out this framework. You don't have to master it overnight. I have seen just a tiny fraction of what I teach here have a profound impact on the lives of our patients.

What I strongly recommend is you take notes as you go through this book. Integrate one or two habits each week. If you can move faster than that, great. This is a marathon, not a sprint.

I picked fourteen days because it's long enough to create a long-term behavior change, but short enough that people don't feel overwhelmed.

I chose the habits for the reset based on my clinical experience. Many of them were inspired by my friend, Jim Laird, who told me that in his experience, three ten-minute walks, a protein at each meal, and plenty of hydration gave his clients the biggest returns on time and effort in their training.

I would implement the habits in the 14-Day Reset before moving on to anything else. You may be tempted to ignore elements of the reset. I recommend you start with the 14-Day Reset and focus on it until you have fully integrated it into your daily life.

I designed the reset to be safe for nearly everyone. That being said, there are rare medical conditions that require us to alter our daily habits. If you have a life-threatening illness, such as cancer, heart, lung, blood, kidney, or liver issues, you should always ask your doctor before making changes to your diet or lifestyle. If you don't have serious medical issues, then this is where I recommend you start your journey through our framework.

When we first built the Reset in our clinic, we included two products we routinely recommend to our patients—a specific light therapy product and blue-blocking glasses. Many of our patients notice faster and better results when they add these.

You do not need any products to start. I have written the Reset so you can begin today with what you already have.

- Start your day with light therapy patches and spend the first five minutes of your day in the brightest sunlight available, without sunglasses or sunscreen (as tolerated—do not burn). If it's too cold outside, find a sunny nook in your home. If it's cloudy or rainy, just find the brightest spot you can. For my favorite light therapy patches, see "Protocols for Energy, Vitality, and Longevity" at stillmanmd.com/autoimmunity.
- Take time to thank, encourage, or compliment at least three people. These positive emotions are powerful healing forces. I tell my wife and son I love them every morning before I leave for work. I send a few texts or emails to employees, colleagues, or friends over coffee. It takes less than sixty seconds, and it will transform your life.
- Take three ten-minute walks, ideally before or immediately after breakfast, lunch, and dinner.
- Drink sixty-four ounces of spring water daily. We will dive deeper into water and hydration later, but for now, make it spring water.
- Each meal needs a cup or a handful of a few key items to cover your essential nutrients. If you don't feel like measuring everything in cups, think of one cup as being the size of your fist.
- Each meal should include:
    - One cup of protein, such as eggs, chicken, turkey, beef, fish, pork, lamb, or bison.
    - One cup of root vegetables, such as potatoes, sweet potatoes, onions, turnips, rutabagas, beets, parsnips, or carrots.
    - One cup of green vegetables, such as cabbage, lettuce, spinach, collards, chard, broccoli, kale, or fennel.
    - One handful of nuts or seeds, such as chia, flax, or pumpkin seeds, walnuts, pecans, pistachios, almonds, hazelnuts, or cashews.

    - Increase these portions if you are highly active.
- At sundown, make your environment as dark as possible. Use low-blue lights. Wear blue blockers if you are around bright lights or are using screens after dark. For more information on these tools and how to use them, see "Protocols for Energy, Vitality, and Longevity" at stillmanmd.com/autoimmunity.
- Get to bed by 10:00 p.m.

The 14-Day Reset is what we start all of our patients with at our practice, because of the profound results that these habits deliver.

These habits aren't exciting, but they are critical to paying down a repair deficit. Small, steady, daily deposits add up faster than you think. Consider the following. When you double a penny every day for thirty days, you end up with over $5 million. If you double it every other day, instead of every day, you end up with $163.84.

Let that sink in.

Consistency pays. A small increase in consistency can lead to a massive increase in results.

Next, we will discuss breathwork, which I consider to be the most important of the essentials.

BREATHWORK: BREATHING TO OPTIMIZE IMMUNITY

"Mouth-breathing youths are sluggards."

—Hippocrates

Dysfunctional breathing mechanics are at the root of many health issues. This has been known for thousands of years.

Yet most people know nothing about breathing mechanics. Most practitioners do not know how to screen for, let alone treat, dysfunctional breathing mechanics.

What are dysfunctional breathing mechanics? They are breathing mechanics that drive dysfunction within the body. Typically, patients take too many breaths that are too shallow and use the wrong muscles to breathe. This is what we call "hyperventilation syndrome."

CARRIE'S STORY: BREATHING GONE WRONG

Carrie came to us after hearing me on a podcast. She had been struggling with panic attacks and anxiety for months. She was losing weight and was concerned she had a serious illness, such as an autoimmune disease. She had been listening to lots of podcasts, all of which gave a different explanation for her illness. Everyone had a supplement, medication, biohack, diet, or lifestyle change for her to try. She felt overwhelmed. She was not sure what to do. She was a full-time working mother. She was expecting a proposal soon from her boyfriend. She felt like her life was finally coming together, and yet she felt like she was coming apart.

I knew within minutes of meeting her that she had dysfunctional breathing mechanics. She was also depleted of minerals and had low progesterone.

After just one month of nutritional supplements and breathwork, she was feeling 70 percent better.

Her initial hair tissue mineral analysis showed depleted levels across the board, indicating chronic exhaustion and nutrient depletion. Four months later, her second test showed dramatic increases in her first four minerals and most trace elements—what we call a "coming alive" pattern. Patients routinely report much more energy, better mood, improved focus and mental clarity, and greater physical stamina with this pattern.

She reported feeling 60–80 percent better within three months of starting our program. She went from having crippling panic attacks and sleeping for only three hours at a time to sleeping six hours and being panic-attack-free.

She gave this breathwork protocol and her personalized supplement protocol 90 percent of the credit for her improvement.

This is why I tell our patients, "You are not allowed to blow off the breathwork." Pun intended.

HYPERVENTILATION SYNDROME

Despite the fact that you may never have heard of it, hyperventilation syndrome is a common problem we face in clinical practice.

Key symptoms include:

- Shortness of breath or feeling unable to get enough air
- Lightheadedness, dizziness, or feeling faint
- Chest pain, tightness, or discomfort
- Rapid, deep, or fast breathing
- Palpitations or a pounding, racing heartbeat
- Numbness or tingling in the hands, feet, or around the mouth
- Muscle spasms or cramps, especially in the hands and feet
- Weakness or confusion
- Sleep disturbances
- Belching, bloating, or dry mouth
- Anxiety, fear, panic, or a sense of impending doom
- Difficulty focusing or thinking clearly
- Frequent sighing or yawning

You take somewhere between 17,000 and 30,000 breaths per day. Every breath you take can pay off your repair deficit, or worsen it. Whenever we see these symptoms, we focus on breathing mechanics first and foremost.

OPTIMAL BREATHING MECHANICS FOR IMMUNE FUNCTION

What do healthy breathing mechanics look like?

First, you should breathe with your diaphragm. This means your chest wall should move in and out with each breath. It should expand both front and back, and on each side. Put your hands on your rib cage. As you breathe in, try to move your hands "out," away from your core. This is circumferential expansion, and it is essential for optimal breathing mechanics.

Second, you should breathe no more than fourteen times per minute on average, based on a fitness tracker. We have long documented in medicine that patients with the fastest respiratory rate have the shortest life expectancy.[15]

Third, most people should breathe through their nose, not their mouth. Short of severe nasal deformities and chronic sinus congestion, you should be able to breathe through your nose. If you can't breathe through your nose, try holding your nose and your breath at the same time, and nodding your head back and forth. This usually triggers your body to clear your nasal passages. If holding your breath is too hard, start with short intervals, but keep going. Most people can relieve nasal congestion with enough of this exercise.

Chronic nasal congestion is often partly due to mouth breathing. Just by increasing the amount of time spent breathing through the nose, many people see their chronic sinus congestion improve or even entirely resolve.

There are rare exceptions to these rules, which is why this is educational information only, not medical advice. Consult a qualified practitioner before engaging in breathwork or changing your breathing mechanics.

BREATHING MECHANICS AND AUTOIMMUNITY

What drives breathing? Most people are surprised to learn that it is carbon dioxide, rather than oxygen.

You breathe when carbon dioxide reaches a certain level in your blood. Carbon dioxide isn't just a waste product of metabolism. It opens your blood vessels and helps oxygen move from the blood into your cells and tissues.

One of the hallmarks of autoimmunity is low tissue oxygen levels and poor blood flow. This is why hyperventilation syndrome keeps close company with autoimmunity.

When we breathe, we also exhale a gas called nitric oxide. Nitric oxide is produced in the nose and sinuses. It opens our blood vessels, like carbon dioxide, and it is an immune signaling molecule. Dysfunction in nitric oxide signaling is strongly linked to autoimmunity.[16]

You can adjust this level by retraining your breathing mechanics. This is life-changing for many people.

Stress, biomechanics, sinus and septum deformities, and nasal congestion drive respiratory mechanics.

Stress triggers the release of hormones and neurotransmitters that cause us to breathe more. Stress is a major contributor to dysfunctional breathing mechanics.

We sit now more than ever before. We move less and less. Even when we do move, it tends to be more repetition than variety. Eventually, people lose mobility in their chest and start taking shallower breaths. To make up for the smaller breaths, people take more breaths. This is a disaster for breathing mechanics.

Nasal deformities and congestion lead to mouth breathing. Your sinuses produce nitric oxide that you need to inhale into your lungs and bloodstream. Nitric oxide lowers blood pressure, modulates the immune system, and improves blood flow. There is a strong association between mouth breathing, obesity, heart disease, and sexual dysfunction.[17] Nitric oxide is the thread that connects them, and its story starts in your nose.

THE STARTING BREATHWORK PROTOCOL

Here's the starting breathwork protocol we share with patients.

We use a metric called "Control Pause," a core concept from Buteyko breathing, to evaluate and monitor breathing mechanics. The Control Pause measures your tolerance to carbon dioxide and helps restore functional breathing mechanics. Our goal is a Control Pause above thirty. Between twenty and thirty is acceptable. Between ten and twenty is a poor prognostic marker. If a patient is below ten, they must increase their control pause if they wish to make progress.

To practice, sit upright, relax, and breathe through your nose. Keep your mouth closed throughout the practice. If you cannot breathe through your nose for any reason, breathe gently through pursed lips as though you were breathing through a straw. Breathe gently through your nose for one minute, focusing on soft, light breaths. Breathe in for three seconds and out for three seconds. This will drop your respiratory rate to ten breaths per minute. You should feel slightly out of breath.

To measure your Control Pause, after a normal exhalation, pinch your nose and hold your breath. Time in seconds how long it takes until you feel the first definite desire to breathe.

Note that this is not as long as possible. This number in seconds is your Control Pause. Release your nose and resume gentle nasal breathing. Take a few recovery breaths. Perform five to ten rounds of the Control Pause within a five-minute session. Between each round, continue gentle nasal breathing.

Do not force the breath hold. Stop at the first urge to breathe. Return to light, silent nasal breathing before and after each Control Pause. Your Control Pause should increase dramatically with this practice. If it does not, we reassess the patient for other factors that may be contributing to dysfunctional breathing mechanics.

We recommend that our patients practice this for at least five minutes, twice daily, morning and evening. Our goal is to increase the Control Pause to twenty to thirty seconds at a minimum. If we have respiratory rate data from some kind of fitness tracker, we will aim for a respiratory rate of under fourteen breaths per minute.

WHAT WE RECOMMEND IN OUR PRACTICE

I will be frank when it comes to the importance of breathing mechanics.

I have learned the hard way that no amount of supplements, drugs, hormones, biohacks, or fancy wellness protocols will make up for dysfunctional breathing mechanics. It is like trying to win a triathlon with a boat anchor tied to both feet.

Usually, the starting breathwork protocol is enough for people. We start patients with twice-daily breathwork and troubleshoot if they do not rapidly improve. Sometimes we send them a more advanced protocol, which is included in the Chapter 3 resources at stillmanmd.com/autoimmunity.

If poor posture or anatomical constraints are impairing

chest-wall expansion, we will refer to our friend Jim Laird, who is a strength and conditioning coach. He has extensive experience helping people optimize their breathing mechanics.

Breathing mechanics are one of the most powerful things we work on with patients, which is why this chapter starts with breathing mechanics.

COMPANION RESOURCES FOR BREATHWORK AND MIND-BODY MEDICINE

The breathwork companion resources at stillmanmd.com/autoimmunity include an advanced protocol for those who want to go deeper, plus guides on mind-body medicine and how we approach allergies.

WATER: HEALING POWER, HIDDEN HAZARDS

"Water is life's matter and matrix, mother and medium; there is no life without water."

—Albert Szent-Gyorgi

Water and hydration are critical for optimal health and immune function. Cellular dehydration is strongly linked to cellular dysfunction, which can manifest as autoimmunity. Water is also a source of nutrients or toxins, depending on its source and how it is treated. Water can worsen your repair deficit or reduce it. You have the power to choose.

Here's a quick story about a patient of ours who was poisoned by their water.

SARAH'S STORY: POISONED BY HER WELL

Sarah came to us in 2024. She had lived on a property with well water some years prior. Unbeknownst to her, the prior property owners had used pesticides for years. There had been industrial activity on the property as well, with unknown metals and chemicals in use. The well casing had cracked. Every time it rained, toxic water seeped into the well.

She underwent chelation therapy for her toxic metal burden at the time. Chelation therapy involves using powerful chemicals classified as drugs to remove heavy metals from the body. She saw great improvements with this, but was convinced she had not eliminated her metal burden.

Her first hair tissue test with us showed remarkable elevations of multiple toxic metals, as well as excess copper and manganese.

Here are her notable heavy metal and mineral levels:

- Lead 276 mcg%
- Cadmium 13 mcg%
- Aluminum 1,550 mcg%
- Nickel 376 mcg%
- Copper 11,800 mcg%
- Manganese 101 mcg%

For reference, our healthiest patients typically have levels that are ten to a hundred times lower than these levels, depending on the metal. These are remarkably abnormal hair tissue results.

We started her on personalized supplements, a new diet, and lifestyle habits.

She reported an improvement in her symptoms of 68 percent by the end of a six-month program at our practice.

WHAT WE RECOMMEND

I have more stories of patients who have been poisoned by their wells or municipal water than I can keep track of. We have a few simple rules and guidelines we share with our patients to protect them from water-borne toxins and to nourish their bodies with proper hydration.

We recommend at least 64 ounces of water daily for optimal hydration. We tailor this to the individual based on their labs and lifestyle. We find that most people need between one and three ounces of water per inch of height—a five foot adult should need no less than 60 ounces, and a six foot five adult should need no more than 231 ounces. These are general rules—there will be unique situations in which they must be broken. You must work with a practitioner to determine optimal hydration for you.

We generally recommend spring or reverse osmosis filtered water.

SPRING WATER

There are three things I like about spring water.

First, it has positively charged minerals like calcium and magnesium. These are vital to good health, and most people are deficient in them. If it is available to you, I strongly recommend magnesium or silica-rich spring water. Most spring water is low in magnesium and silica.

Second, certain spring waters contain silica. Silica is the antidote to aluminum, which is a major driver of autoimmunity.

Third, water is programmed by the electromagnetic forces of nature. This has been well-established by scientists like Gerald Pollack, PhD, editor of the journal *Water*. This has subtle but marked effects on our health and well-being. We recommend spring water because it is programmed by the electromagnetic field of the earth, and nothing else.

FILTERED AND DISTILLED WATER

If you are drinking well or municipal water, then I strongly recommend that you test and filter or distill it. We see cases of well or municipal water poisoning every year in our practice. In most cases, patients have a water filter. They wrongly assume this protects them from toxins in their water. People often choose the wrong filter, or the contaminants in their water overwhelm the filter.

If you decide to use reverse osmosis or distilled water, I suggest taking a daily mineral supplement to compensate for the effects of reverse osmosis or distilled water on your mineral balance. Reverse osmosis and distilled water pull minerals out of the body. I cover this in more detail in the companion resources.

WHAT WE RECOMMEND AGAINST

If it's not reverse osmosis, distilled, or spring water, I can't recommend it. Many companies claim to filter various contaminants, particularly fluoride. I do not believe their claims. I have seen third-party evidence proving many of these claims to be false.

AVOID PLASTIC WHENEVER POSSIBLE

Avoid plastic whenever possible. Sometimes, it isn't practical. For the record, I have spent years drinking water out of five-gallon plastic bottles. Why did I do that, when I recommend against plastic? Because I didn't have the option of glass bottled water delivery in my location at the time. You might. Glass might not be practical for you, for many reasons.

It is not a perfect world. Your water won't be perfect either, and that's okay. Don't lose sleep over the imperfections of your water. You don't have to sell all your worldly possessions and set up camp by your nearest artisanal spring. Just pick a reasonable solution and improve upon it when and how you can.

Your body is either paying down its repair deficit with every glass of water you drink, or your repair deficit is worsening. You consume thousands of liters of water each year, between what you drink and what you cook with. We have to fix our water and optimize our hydration to resolve a repair deficit. This is why, after breathing, we tackle water and hydration.

COMPANION RESOURCES FOR WATER AND HYDRATION

I have more to share with you on this topic. The water companion resources at stillmanmd.com/autoimmunity include guides for testing and filtering your water, silica-rich water for aluminum detoxification, and electrolyte formulas. If you're curious to know what water filters I recommend, and my most important advice about water and hydration, check out "Healing Waters: Hydration to Nourish, Detoxify, and Repair."

SUNLIGHT: THE FORGOTTEN HEALER

"Mal-illumination is to light what malnutrition is to food."

—John Ott

Sunlight is one of our most powerful healers. The oath physicians took in ancient Greece, the Hippocratic Oath, historically began with the words, "I swear to Apollo the healer." Apollo was the Greek god of healing and the sun. Despite this, modern medicine has forgotten how powerful a healer the sun truly is.

As we move further and further from the equator, we get less and less sun during the year. As we move further and further from the equator, we also see the incidence and severity of autoimmunity rise.[18]

This is not a coincidence. The sun is a powerful protector of the immune system. If I had to give you a single analogy, sunlight "modulates" your immune system to tolerate your cells and tissues, while attacking what it should attack: pathogens, toxins, cancerous cells, and so on.

What does this mean? The more sun you get, the lower your risk of autoimmunity. The less sun you get, the greater your risk of autoimmunity.

Working nights and evenings usually means getting less sun during the day, but it also means exposure to artificial light at night. This is why working at night is strongly linked to autoimmunity.[19]

The healing power of sunlight is why the 14-Day Reset includes three ten-minute walks. This is why the reset also includes a strict bedtime to help you get up and spend more time in sunlight.

Many patients with autoimmunity notice they cannot tolerate strong light. Patients may have light-sensitive headaches. They may develop terrible skin rashes if exposed to too much sunlight. We call this photosensitivity. You should consult a qualified practitioner about how much sun to get, because there are cases in which we have to be careful with the dose.

Most of all, avoid getting sunburned. Sunburn increases your risk of skin cancer and ages your skin.

For most patients, more sunlight is better. Here is a quick story to illustrate the power of the sun.

ASHLEE'S STORY: LIGHT FOR THYROID AND JOINT HEALTH

Ashlee Rowland grew up in Alaska and was diagnosed at fourteen years old with rheumatoid arthritis, Hashimoto's thyroiditis, and severe acne. She was told this was just how life was going to be for her. Nothing else could be done.

She accepted this at first, not knowing any better, but life led her to people who knew better. Through friends and family, she was introduced to many of the ideas in this book.

Ashlee reinvented her life and restored her health. Years after her initial diagnosis, she happened to move to Hawaii to be a nanny. The family she lived with ate healthy food, spent plenty of time at the beach, and otherwise lived a healthy lifestyle. Her skin symptoms cleared, her joint pain resolved, and her energy returned—all within weeks of arriving in Hawaii. She was shocked.

Ashlee and I have recorded three podcasts about her journey. In part one, we cover her recovery in Hawaii. In part two, we cover her journey to restoring her fertility and having her first child. In part three, we cover her family's experience with mold and how it nearly undid everything. All three are worth your time.

Hear Ashlee's story at stillmanmd.com/autoimmunity.

We hear stories like Ashlee's on a regular basis at our practice.

WHAT WE RECOMMEND IN OUR PRACTICE

Sunlight consists of infrared light, visible light, and ultraviolet light. Infrared and red light, in particular, help our bodies to repair. We need daily infrared and red light for optimal health and immunity. Sunlight is approximately 42 percent infrared light.[20] Your average fluorescent bulb or LED emits zero infrared light. Most people now spend more than 90 percent of their lives indoors or in their vehicles.[21] Our infrared light exposure has effectively gone to zero in just a few generations. Ultraviolet light has been known to treat autoimmune diseases for over one hundred years.[22] We still use it in our practice. We will cover light therapy in Chapter 6 and in the companion resources at stillmanmd.com/autoimmunity.

We recommend that patients get as much sun exposure as possible, while carefully avoiding sunburns or other side effects of intense light (such as headaches or skin rashes). We start patients with three ten-minute walks as part of the 14-Day Reset. We strongly recommend spending your day, whether indoors or outdoors, in natural light. Sit near a window. Keep the blinds open. Wear sunglasses, hats, and sunscreen only if you truly need them.

What about skin cancer? Dermatologists have told the public to fear the sun, but as we will cover in the next chapter, this may have done more harm than good.

Every hour you spend under artificial light is an hour your body misses out on the benefits of natural light. Not long ago, we spent 100 percent of our time in natural light. Today, it might be less than 2 or 3 percent of our time. Sunlight is a powerful healer. Can you resolve a repair deficit without it? Perhaps, but I would not count on it. This is why we prioritize getting outside every single day.

COMPANION RESOURCES FOR LIGHT AND HEALTH

The companion resources at stillmanmd.com/autoimmunity include our complete light therapy protocols for red, infrared, and UV light, plus sauna therapy guidance and Ashlee's three-part podcast about her recovery.

FOOD: NUTRITION OR TRIGGER

"Let thy food be thy medicine."

—Hippocrates

Food is one of the main drivers of autoimmunity today. This is due to contamination with pesticides, hormones, and toxins like mercury. Many of us believe that genetic modification of food is playing a role as well.

Patients hear stories about food and autoimmunity, and often feel lost as to what to do with the information.

I have seen countless testimonials of autoimmune diseases going into remission practically overnight when the patient eliminated a certain food or started a restrictive diet.

This begs more questions than it answers. What should you eat? What should you stop eating? Should you base these decisions on lab testing? Should you stop eating gluten? Dairy? What about goat or sheep dairy? Nightshades? Grains? Pseudograins?

We keep things simple. Here is our approach.

As your body accumulates toxins and is exposed to more and more stress, your body starts to lose immune tolerance to anything and everything. "Immune tolerance" is the technical term for "not attacking things." If your immune system tolerates gluten, then you can eat gluten and your body will digest it. If your immune system loses tolerance to gluten, your body will attack it.

Immune reactions driven by food can vary from person to person. This is a major source of confusion for practitioners and patients alike.

Here is a quick case study from our practice.

MARY'S STORY: HIDDEN INGREDIENTS DRIVING GUT DYSFUNCTION

Mary came to us with crippling abdominal pain. She could not figure out what was causing it. She had seen many doctors and tried everything she could think of. Her children were in college, and one of her greatest joys in life was traveling to see them. She felt like her gut issues were derailing her life.

We ran food allergy testing. She tested positive for corn. Corn is used to manufacture a huge proportion of the food additives used in the United States. When she eliminated corn, she experienced a 90 percent improvement in her abdominal pain. She was able to leave the house again. She was able to travel and, more importantly to her, be present for her family. She went from worrying about where her symptoms were going to functioning at her best on a daily basis.

Food plays a major role in autoimmunity. Mary's case is one of many like it from our practice.

In conventional medicine, the dogma is that environmental exposures and foods do not cause autoimmune diseases. The problem with this theory is that it is not supported by the facts. Reports of patients achieving remission from autoimmunity by eliminating triggers from their diet, personal care products, or environment are widespread. These patients clearly demonstrate a causal relationship between exposure and symptoms.

Do not be fooled by the conventional dogma. Whatever you want to call them—allergies, allergic triggers, autoimmune triggers—there is no denying that what you are exposed to in your environment can drive autoimmunity. From the perfume or cologne you spray on your body in the morning to what you eat for breakfast, lunch, or dinner to your organic spearmint toothpaste that you brush your teeth with before you go to bed, anything can become a trigger for autoimmunity. It follows that we can induce remission of autoimmunity by eliminating these allergic triggers from our environments. This is what we see in practice.

WHAT WE RECOMMEND AT OUR PRACTICE

We try to keep things simple at our practice. Here is what we share with our patients.

We tell all of them to stop eating gluten, dairy, fried foods, and processed sugar. There are two reasons for this. First, they may actually have lost immune tolerance to these foods. Second, if you eliminate these foods, you have eliminated 90 percent of processed foods. Processed foods drive all types of disease, including autoimmunity. The more processed food you eat, the sicker you will become and the shorter your life will be.[23]

Most of our patients have already eliminated some or all of these foods, or at least are moderating their consumption of them.

Many of our patients have already gone to some kind of extreme in their diet. I have seen every kind of diet work. Whether or not they are sustainable is another matter. We often see patients who long to eat more than just a few foods or food groups. We do our best to help them regain tolerance to foods they are allergic to or intolerant of.

We often recommend allergy testing to identify triggers of autoimmunity. If testing is not an option, we recommend systematic elimination of foods and ingredients to sort out what a patient's triggers are.

When allergy testing is positive, it is often life-changing. Patients often report 90 percent or better improvement with the elimination of the offending triggers alone. On the other hand, many patients see no appreciable difference. This is frequently because they have not eliminated the foods they are allergic to. They are hidden ingredients in processed foods that people are still eating.

We will cover allergy testing later. I have practiced with and without allergy testing. We can still get great results without it, but there are cases in which it is invaluable.

You eat three or more times a day, over a thousand meals a year. Each meal either feeds repair or feeds a repair deficit. There is no neutral. This is why food is one of the essentials we address early and often.

COMPANION RESOURCES FOR FOOD

The companion resources at stillmanmd.com/autoimmunity include meal plans, a simple diet assessment tool, guidance on fasting and meal timing, and our Fish, Fish Oil, and Autoimmunity Guide.

EXERCISE: RESTORATIVE OR DESTRUCTIVE

"Walking is a man's best medicine."

—Hippocrates

Exercise has a complex relationship with autoimmunity. Exercise is a form of stress. There are two different types of stress—eustress and distress. Eustress is stress that your body can handle and adapt to. Eustress is what gives us bigger muscles, faster reflexes, better coordinated movements, and greater stamina. Distress is stress that overwhelms your system and your ability to adapt. Distress leads to muscle wasting, exhaustion, over-training syndrome, and burnout.

Eustress is healthy. Distress creates disease. The key is knowing the difference.

No one knows the difference better than my friend, Jim Laird.

JIM'S STORY: POWERLIFTING AND ULCERATIVE COLITIS

Jim Laird is a strength and conditioning coach with over two decades of experience. He was setting world records in powerlifting when he suddenly developed ulcerative colitis, an autoimmune disorder that affects the colon and causes severe and sometimes life-threatening bleeding.

He discovered that exercise was part of his problem. He restricted his diet as we described in the prior section, added targeted supplements and over-the-counter medications, and dealt with the anger that was one of the emotional causes of his illness. He has been symptom-free with no medications for over ten years. Today, he educates high performers about the dangers of pushing themselves so hard that they develop autoimmunity.

Jim and I recorded a podcast about his story in two parts. In part one, we cover his experience with ulcerative colitis. In part two, we cover the chronic infections that showed up years later. If you push yourself hard physically, this one's for you. Hear Jim's story at stillmanmd.com/autoimmunity.

WHAT WE RECOMMEND IN OUR PRACTICE

Generally, we recommend that patients seeking to recover from autoimmunity restrict exercise to light weightlifting and walking three times daily for ten minutes. More is often a liability.

I always return to the concept of a repair deficit when thinking about autoimmunity. Your body is always trying to repair itself. It only has so many resources to meet your needs for repair. If your body is constantly using its resources to fix the damage from exercise, you can slow or even stop your healing entirely.

This is why we start most of our patients on just three ten-minute walks each day. These are not "power" walks. They are slow, relaxed walks. Jim came up with this habit, and we have kept it ever since he introduced it to us. These walks are powerfully restorative. As patients recover their health, we can introduce more and higher intensity exercise to accelerate their healing.

I counsel patients to find a good trainer. Whether you call them a coach, personal trainer, or health coach, find someone to hold you accountable to moving your body every day.

Exercise can accelerate repair or deepen a repair deficit. It depends on the dose, duration, and intensity of exercise. Too much exercise is one of the most overlooked causes of a repair deficit that we see in practice. This is why we start with walking, not intense exercise.

COMPANION RESOURCES FOR EXERCISE

The companion resources at stillmanmd.com/autoimmunity include Jim's two-part podcast about his recovery from ulcerative colitis and our guide to exercising without creating a repair deficit.

ESSENTIALS: THE ROOTS OF GOOD HEALTH

I think of health as being like a tree. Good habits—the essentials—are like the roots of the tree. Without them, the tree falls over. I start with them because I expect patients who ignore them to fail, no matter how hard we try, no matter how much money we spend, and no matter how much we hope they will recover.

The patients whose stories you've read in this book all did the essentials. That's part of why they achieved exceptional results.

Many people dismiss the essentials because they think of them as inconsequential. Do not make that mistake. The essentials, done consistently enough for long enough, often deliver better results than complicated, expensive medical procedures or protocols. This is why we start with the essentials.

YOUR NEXT STEP

You now have the five essentials that form the foundation of healing. Start with the 14-Day Reset tomorrow morning. If you have serious medical issues, such as heart, lung, kidney, liver, or blood issues, consult your physician before implementing the essentials. There are rare cases where these choices will not be right for you.

Take the Repair Deficit Survey every two weeks at stillmanmd.com/autoimmunity. As you build the essentials into your routine, watch how your score changes. Healing is not linear—some symptoms may worsen before they improve, and scores sometimes rise before they fall. This is normal. Your score over time tells you whether you're heading in the right direction.

There is so much more for me to share with you about the essentials. Download the companion resources for each essential at stillmanmd.com/autoimmunity.

You can submit questions for our Q&A shows at stillmanmd.com/autoimmunity.

The essentials build your foundation, like the roots of a

tree. But no matter how deep and strong your roots are, they are vulnerable. If you aren't careful, all the hard work you put into the essentials will be undermined by toxins and stresses in your diet, lifestyle, and environment. We call these toxins and stresses "Hazards." These are things you must remove or avoid for optimal health and immunity.

COMPANION RESOURCES FOR CHAPTER 3

The Chapter 3 companion resources at stillmanmd.com/autoimmunity bring together everything you need to go deeper on the essentials. You will find:

- Breathing guides, including an advanced protocol and our guide to mind-body medicine
- Guides to hydration, water filters, and more
- Guides to meal planning, assessing your diet, and more
- Podcasts with Ashlee and Jim about the power of the essentials for healing

You can submit questions about the essentials for our Q&A shows at stillmanmd.com/autoimmunity.

CHAPTER 4

Hazards

"Before seeking to heal anyone, ask him if he is willing to give up what is making him sick."

—HIPPOCRATES

The body cannot repair itself when it is exposed to more toxins and stressors than it can handle. These are the "Hazards" of modern life. In this chapter, we explore the Hazards that have the greatest impact on our patients with autoimmunity. You may be surprised by what made the list. This chapter is not based on theory. It is based on real-world experience.

Autoimmunity is increasing in prevalence and severity due to Hazards in our modern world. These include habits and lifestyle choices, exposures to toxic chemicals, and trauma from toxic relationships. In this chapter, we will explore what these things are, how they create a repair deficit, and how to avoid them.

We have already touched on several of them in previous chapters. These include processed food, artificial light, chemicals like pesticides and herbicides, heavy metals, and more.

Many Hazards that drive autoimmunity are things that people struggle to give up, like their favorite foods, drugs, activities, or creature comforts. The patients who do best tend to be the strictest about avoiding the Hazards of modern life that create a repair deficit.

This is not an exhaustive guide to this topic. That would be a book in itself. This is an overview of what you most need to know to protect yourself and your family.

THE 14-DAY DETOX

Before we dive into why each Hazard matters, let me give you the action plan. This is where everyone starts. If you need product recommendations to make this happen, "Protocols for Energy, Vitality, and Longevity" is where you will find them.

Five simple swaps will eliminate the most important sources of toxic exposure and stress in your daily life. Start today. Track for fourteen days. Notice what changes.

1. Eliminate aluminum. Switch to aluminum-free deodorant. Eliminate all aluminum-canned beverages, including energy drinks, sodas, and beer. Check your labels. Many baking powders contain aluminum. Check your medications for aluminum and ask your doctor about aluminum-free alternatives.
2. Swap out toxic sunscreens for zinc oxide sunscreen. Replace all other types of sunscreen. Consider the importance of daily sun exposure, as we covered in Chapter 3.
3. Minimize light and electronics in your bedroom. Use blackout curtains, blinds, or drapes to make your bedroom as dark as possible. Turn off or unplug Wi-Fi, Bluetooth, and any other wireless emitters or transmitters in your bedroom

nightly. Put your phone on airplane mode or leave it in another room. If you can't turn these things off, place them as far from where you sleep as possible. Sleep as far from smart meters as possible (twenty feet is a bare minimum in our practice).

4. Eliminate mercury-rich fish. This means no tuna, swordfish, shark, mahi, seabass, grouper, or king mackerel. If you aren't sure about a fish, look it up (we have a guide to Fish, Fish Oil, and Autoimmunity, where we cover this). Switch to low-mercury options like wild salmon, sardines, anchovies, and herring. If you eat fish multiple times per week, this matters immensely.
5. Stop smoking and vaping. Switch to alternative forms if you are using substances medicinally. Seek to wean off if you are addicted. Inhalation is the fastest route to your bloodstream and to chronic illness.

Track your symptoms daily for fourteen days. Some people notice changes within days or weeks. Some see dramatic improvements. Others notice subtle shifts in sleep quality, mental clarity, energy levels, or pain.

COMPANION RESOURCES FOR THE 14-DAY DETOX

Product recommendations to make this happen can be found in "Protocols for Energy, Vitality, and Longevity," at stillmanmd.com/autoimmunity.

Now let me show you why each of these swaps matters.

ALUMINUM: A HIDDEN CAUSE OF AUTOIMMUNITY

"Human exposure to aluminium is the yet unrecognised, unprecedented threat to the future of mankind."

—Dr. Christopher Exley, PhD, FRS

Aluminum is everywhere. Most baking soda contains aluminum. Most underarm deodorants contain aluminum. Most vaccines contain aluminum. Many processed foods are packaged in aluminum. Energy drinks, sodas, and beer come in aluminum cans. You'll find it in spice and herb blends. Kids' snack and juice pouches are lined with aluminum. I even hear reports of people finding aluminum in their soil from geoengineering.

Aluminum is toxic in any quantity. It is not as acutely toxic as mercury, cadmium, lead, or arsenic, which is why regulatory bodies consider it "safe." This is nonsense. It just isn't as toxic as mercury, which is lethal even in tiny doses. Aluminum is a major driver of autoimmunity, among other diseases, in our modern world.[24]

It is clearly implicated in autoimmunity, though vested corporate interests are fighting this narrative tooth and nail to preserve their profits. Here's a story about the clinical reality of aluminum toxicity and autoimmunity we see daily in our practice.

TERESA'S STORY: ALUMINUM, SUNSCREEN, AND SCLERODERMA

Teresa contacted me when she was diagnosed with scleroderma, a rare autoimmune condition of the skin. Scleroderma is one of those diseases doctors are terrified of. The disease causes skin all over the body to form scars. These scars restrict blood flow to the extremities. Patients eventually lose fingers and toes due to a lack of blood flow. Their faces become frozen as their skin scars down. As this happens, they gradually lose the ability to open their mouths. Ultimately, they lose the ability to speak and to eat. Conventional treatments do not work. Patients are given little, if any hope, by the conventional medical system.

Teresa lived in the Upper Midwest. Her dermatologist told her to wear sunscreen and never let the sun touch her skin or her eyes. Teresa was wearing sunscreen and sunglasses as she commuted in her car. Car windows and windshields block 100 percent of UV light. This advice makes no sense whatsoever. Teresa had zero exposure to UV light on a day-to-day basis. She wasted her time and money on her dermatologist-recommended skincare routine. It's like wearing a rain jacket and waterproof boots every day in the deserts of Arizona or New Mexico, or a fur coat and hat in Florida.

Teresa's sunscreen contained aluminum. I told her to stop using it immediately. She stopped wearing her sunglasses too. She started getting as much sun as she could. She changed her diet. She embraced the essentials from Chapter 3.

Her disease went into remission. She went from having one of the most feared diagnoses in medicine to good health virtually overnight. Individual results vary, of course, but this story impressed upon me just how dangerous aluminum can be.

For the first several years of my practice, I did not test aluminum levels, and I knew little about aluminum toxicology. Then I started to measure aluminum levels in hair. Emily's case (Chapter 2) was one of the first where I saw a massive metal elimination coincide with a significant clinical improvement. I was convinced thereafter. Few practitioners today test a patient for aluminum for many reasons. The more I tested aluminum in my patients, the more concerned I became.

The record for hair aluminum in our practice is that of an

entrepreneur who was using energy drinks to drive performance. His aluminum level was 134,000 mcg%. Most of our patients consume no aluminum-containing products, and their levels are under 2,000 mcg%. I am convinced that aluminum is driving many of our epidemics of chronic disease, not just autoimmunity. I believe it is driving the epidemics of neurodegenerative disease (dementia, particularly Alzheimer's), allergy, metabolic disorders, heart disease, and more.[25] These are topics for future books.

ALUMINUM AVOIDANCE

Aluminum is found in personal care products, foods, food additives, and culinary ingredients (like baking soda), sunscreen, and more. Anything packaged in aluminum cans or pouches is likely contaminated with high levels of aluminum. Dry goods (powders and dried fruit, for example) are likely not contaminated. Avoid aluminum. For more information on aluminum detoxification, check out the companion resources at stillmanmd.com/autoimmunity.

MERCURY: THE MOST TOXIC HEAVY METAL

"The dose makes the poison."

—Paracelsus

Mercury is toxic in any dose. It has been used in medicine and dentistry for centuries, despite abundant evidence that it causes harm even in small doses. Dentists are still taught that mercury is safe, and many still use mercury amalgam to fill cavities. They have done incalculable harm to humanity in their stubborn refusal to acknowledge that mercury, in any dose or form, is toxic to life. Much of the mercury in our environment, which is poisoning our ecosystems, has been put there by dentists.

RICHARD'S STORY: MERCURY TOXICITY AND GRAVES' DISEASE

Richard was referred to me by his brother. He called me in May 2024 when his symptoms of Graves' disease (autoimmune hyperthyroidism) returned. Years before, he had been evaluated by the Mayo Clinic for the same problem. They had recommended a thyroidectomy (the removal of the thyroid gland). He had ignored them and gone to an integrative practitioner, who treated him for Lyme disease. He went into remission and had avoided doctors ever since.

Lab testing confirmed hyperthyroidism and also revealed a low cortisol level. Cortisol is a hormone that regulates our energy, metabolism, and immune systems. Low levels are common in patients with autoimmunity.

I immediately prescribed a trio of medications we routinely use to treat hyperthyroidism—propranolol, methimazole, and prednisone. We used low doses, and his symptoms quickly abated.

He also had elevated levels of mercury, aluminum, and copper in his hair. He had an unusually high omega-3 index for someone who did not take fish oil supplements. I asked him about the mercury and high omega-3 levels. High-mercury fish like tuna, swordfish, and sea bass were his favorite foods to order at fine restaurants. He cut out fish from his diet and stuck to red meat instead.

We started him on a personalized supplement protocol. We added high-dose vitamin C and light therapy patches.

Just a few months later, we stopped all of his thyroid medications, and he has remained well ever since. His thyroid hormone numbers are within normal ranges. Far from needing a thyroidectomy, he just needed to address the toxins that were driving his hyperthyroidism.

MERCURY AVOIDANCE

Mercury, unfortunately, is now found throughout our environment. Trace amounts are present in practically everything, including food and water. Mercury accumulates in predators, particularly in the ocean. This means that the larger the fish, the higher the mercury levels (as a general rule).

Avoid tuna of all types, swordfish, shark, king mackerel, sea bass, and halibut. Can you have the occasional tuna roll or swordfish steak? The sicker the patient, the more carefully they must avoid mercury. I would only allow the occasional (once monthly) indulgence of high-mercury fish even in a robust and entirely healthy patient.

I recommend that people eat fish or take fish oil to optimize their omega-3 fatty acid levels. Safe options include wild salmon, sardines, anchovies, herring, and Atlantic mackerel (not King mackerel). For more information on this topic, check out "Fish, Fish Oil, and Autoimmunity" in the companion resources.

Under no circumstances should anyone ever receive mercury amalgam fillings. I have many more case studies like this one. There are few topics I feel more strongly about.

For those of you who have mercury fillings, I strongly recommend consultation with a biological dentist who is properly trained in mercury amalgam removal. For recommendations on dentists and other practitioners, go to stillmanmd.com/autoimmunity and look for the companion resource, "Good Dentistry: Healthy Teeth for Life."

CHEMICAL SUNSCREENS: MORE HARM THAN GOOD

"The sun is the best physician."

—Auguste Rollier, MD

The more sun you get, the longer you will live. This was the critical finding of the Melanoma in Southern Sweden Study, one of the greatest studies ever done on the effects of sun exposure.[26] Melanoma is the most feared form of skin cancer. Approximately eight thousand Americans die from melanoma each year, and many more are disfigured. Survivors live in fear of having to undergo surgery again and again for recurrence. It is a terrible illness that has been entirely blamed on the sun.

However, I would argue that blaming the sun for melanoma is like blaming spoons for our obesity epidemic. The facts tell a different story. Did you know that melanoma patients who get the most sun exposure live the longest?[27] Read that again and think about it for a moment. If the sun causes melanoma, then why do melanoma patients who get the least sun have the highest risk of death? Electrical line workers, who work outside year-round for decades, have a higher risk of skin cancer than the general public, but not a higher risk of melanoma. How is this possible if the sun causes melanoma? If the sun causes skin cancer, why do skin cancer rates double every few decades, while sun exposure has decreased to record lows and sunscreen use is at record highs?

The answer, at least in part, lies in the toxic nature of modern sunscreens. Sunscreens have not been proven to prevent melanoma, the most deadly skin cancer.[28] Sunscreen use has even been linked in some studies to an increased risk of death by melanoma.[29] Sunscreens are so toxic that they are banned at many nature preserves and parks because they can cause severe damage to delicate ecosystems. If they are toxic to aquatic ecosystems, why would they be safe for you?

Teresa's story demonstrates this perfectly. Her aluminum-containing sunscreen was poisoning her. Once she eliminated it and restored natural sun exposure, she saw transformational results.

Sunburns have been tied to skin cancer, so we should avoid getting sunburned. Our recommendations to patients to protect their skin are to cover up, use zinc oxide sunscreen, or get under shade if they cannot stand more sun.

I use sunglasses when I am on the water, in the snow, or driving in extremely bright conditions. Otherwise, I let sunlight hit my eyes unimpeded. If I am squinting, I will reach for a hat first, then sunglasses, and rarely both. Patients frequently tell me they start to feel better with this simple change to their daily routine.

ELECTROMAGNETIC POLLUTION: THE INVISIBLE TOXIN

"The greatest polluting element in the earth's environment is the proliferation of electromagnetic fields."

—Robert O. Becker, MD

The electromagnetic force is one of the fundamental forces of nature. You use it every day when you turn on and use household appliances, make phone calls or send text messages from your cell phone, use any smart device, or even just start your car. Over the last hundred years, our electromagnetic environment has changed radically. We have introduced what I will call "electrosmog"—electromagnetic fields and energies that are harmful to life.

Patients often experience profound healing when they eliminate sources of electrosmog in their daily lives. Here is a story from our practice about what's possible.

KELLY'S STORY: HASHIMOTO'S, HEADACHES, AND ELECTROSMOG

Kelly had been struggling with Hashimoto's, fibromyalgia, and severe headaches for years. She had "tried everything." Her headaches were so severe that she was not sure how to live with them any longer. She was busy helping her husband run their medical practice and parenting her daughter through the challenges and temptations of college. In addition to personalized supplements based on lab testing, I strongly urged her to have her home inspected for electrosmog.

What she found astonished her. Her house was inundated by electrosmog. Her headaches went from an 11/10 before to a 7/10 after nutritional supplements and lifestyle changes, but the electrosmog mitigation took them from 7/10 to 4/10. She was thrilled.

Patients who take their electromagnetic environment seriously often get the best results of all of our patients.

WHAT WE RECOMMEND IN OUR PRACTICE

The hardest thing about dealing with electrosmog is that it is increasingly a part of daily life. Minimizing exposure takes time and effort, but it turns out to be one of the highest-yield interventions that our patients make.

Start with the low-hanging fruit in the 14-Day Detox. That is enough for most patients to see profound improvements in sleep, energy, and cognitive function, among other things. You'll find more information in the companion resource, "What's in Your Home That's Confusing Your Immune System?"

If you would like to learn more about the effects of electrosmog on human health, listen to my podcast with Dr. Olle Johansson. He is one of the world's foremost experts on this topic. If you're skeptical about electrosmog and health, start there.

I also interviewed Loredo Ritter, MD, about his work studying the effects of electrosmog on sleep and health. He is a pediatric neurologist who now assesses electromagnetic fields in people's homes. This is one of my favorite podcasts—especially the discussion on children and sleep.

You will find all of the companion resources at stillmanmd.com/autoimmunity.

SMOKING AND VAPING: DIRECT DELIVERY TO THE BLOODSTREAM

"It's important for the FDA, the e-cigarette companies and vapers themselves to know that these heating coils, as currently made, seem to be leaking toxic metals—which then get into the aerosols that vapers inhale."

—Ana María Rule, PhD, Johns Hopkins Bloomberg School of Public Health

I am strongly opposed to any kind of smoked, vaporized, or nebulized recreational drug use. Some of our toughest cases in the practice fell ill while smoking or vaping recreational drugs. Inhalation is the best way to get chemicals into your body and the fastest way to poison yourself.

JAMES'S STORY: VAPING AND LYMPHOCYTIC COLITIS

James was in his early twenties when he came to see me. He is a social media influencer who developed severe diarrhea. His formal diagnosis was lymphocytic colitis. Nothing would stop it. He finally went carnivore, and the crippling stomach pain and liquid stools finally stopped. As soon as he ate anything other than meat, his symptoms returned.

We tried everything. When I say that we tried everything, I mean I shared every single tool and tactic in this entire book with James, plus many of the more advanced protocols we cover in the companion resources online, and he still required high doses of immunosuppressants to remain symptom-free. He is one of the only patients to go through our autoimmunity program and report zero improvement in the first three months. He finally found some relief with medications.

I am still actively working on the case. I am still optimistic we can help him lead a normal life.

What was different about James? He was vaping regularly. Inhalation bypasses all of the body's protective barriers. Whatever you inhale goes directly into your bloodstream and then throughout your entire body. This includes your brain, your organs, and your immune system.

Please do not vape or smoke. It is not worth it.

If you are using these substances medicinally or are addicted, I understand. Switch to alternative forms, such as edibles, tinctures, or pills. Seek to wean off as you are able. Your body will thank you.

OTHER COMMON HAZARDS

Beyond the five swaps in the 14-Day Detox, other hazards are worth mentioning briefly.

Fluoride is in toothpaste and tap water. Because it is in tap water, it winds up in processed food and bottled beverages. Fluoride is a toxin known to poison every system of the body, and particularly to lower your intelligence (based on IQ scores).[30] This is why we took it out of the water in Florida. The only type of filter I trust to remove fluoride is a reverse osmosis filter. This is why we recommend spring water or reverse osmosis filtered water.

Processed food is full of toxic preservatives, colorings, flavorings, and more. Many of these ingredients are linked to autoimmunity. If it comes in a box, bottle, bag, or glass or plastic container, then it is processed. Unprocessed food comes from the butcher case and the produce section. The sicker the patient, the more important it is for them to eat unprocessed food. This is why the 14-Day Reset meal plan includes only whole foods that are easy to prepare by boiling, sautéing, or roasting.

Artificial light at night is a major cause of autoimmunity. Shift work (working at night) is well-known to be associated with higher rates of autoimmune diseases. This is why we recommend blue blockers and a strict bedtime in the 14-Day Reset, and darkening your bedroom at night in the 14-Day Detox.

Toxic personal care products are everywhere. We routinely recommend that patients cut back their personal care products to nothing for a few weeks—not even toothpaste or soap, just water. You would be shocked at some of the stories I hear when patients quit using their personal care products.

Synthetic clothing is made with toxic chemicals. These chemicals might not bother your nose, but they are slowly suffusing into your body via your skin. More than one woman in my practice has told me that upon switching to natural clothing, particularly cotton or wool underwear, numerous health issues disappeared.

Frequent travel is one of the greatest stresses of modern life. Our jet-setting, travel-happy patients are often the toughest cases. You can travel, just do so in moderation.

WHEN PRODUCTS POISON YOU

For the skeptics, here are three different hair tests from three different men, all using the same hair product. Their lead levels are certainly due to product contamination. We do not see levels this high unless it is being directly applied to the hair. One of these patients had significant elevations in his blood, proving he was truly poisoned by this product. Two independent labs tested the product he had been using, and both confirmed the product had high concentrations of lead.

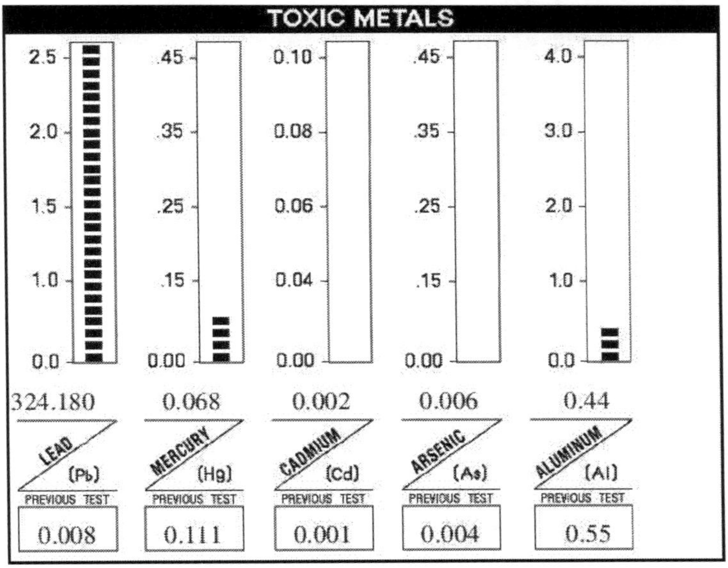

Figure 3. Elevated lead from a hair-loss product, patient A

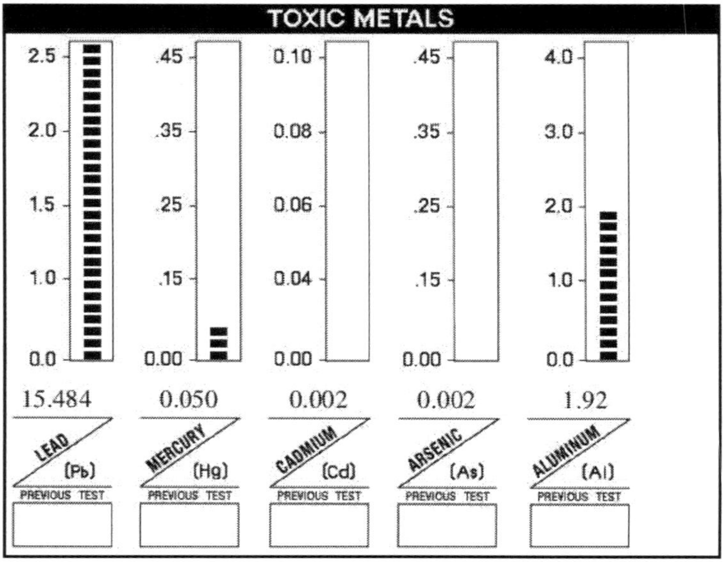

Figure 4. Elevated lead from a hair-loss product, patient B

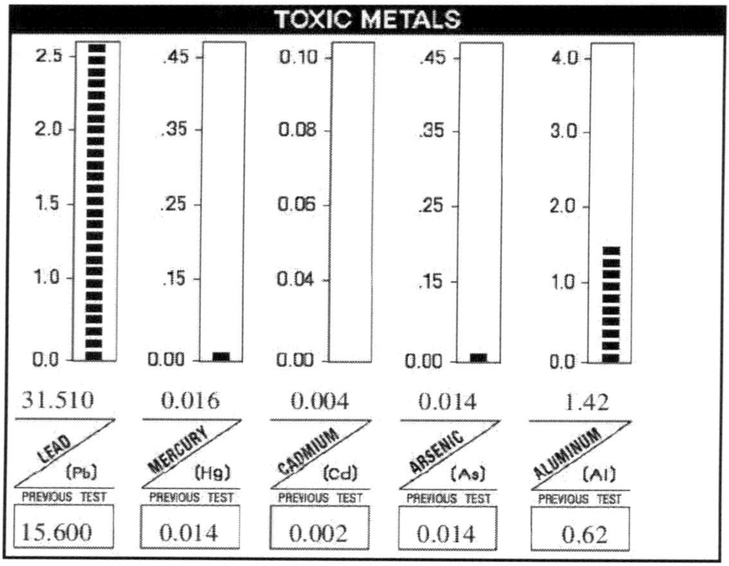

Figure 5. Elevated lead from a hair-loss product, patient C

I have more case studies on contaminated consumer products than I could include here. I share more of them in the companion resources section online.

COMPANION RESOURCES FOR HAZARDS

The companion resources at stillmanmd.com/autoimmunity include guides on how to avoid these common hazards in food, clothing, personal care products, and your home. You will also find case studies of contaminated products there.

Next, we have to discuss a difficult and increasingly common cause of autoimmunity—modern medicine.

DRUGS, VACCINES, AND AUTOIMMUNITY: WHEN MEDICINE MAKES YOU SICK

"One of the first duties of the physician is to educate the masses not to take medicine."

—Sir William Osler, MD

Drugs and vaccines are well-known to cause autoimmunity. Drug-induced autoimmunity is a common occurrence, and anyone who develops an autoimmune disease should take a good, hard look at their medication list.[31] We aggressively de-prescribe, that is, eliminate medications at our practice to avoid any possibility of drug-induced autoimmunity.

DRUG-INDUCED AUTOIMMUNITY

Some drugs are more likely to cause autoimmunity than others, but we treat all of them as guilty until proven innocent.

A few years ago, I would have included a comprehensive list of drugs that cause autoimmunity. Instead, I am giving you an AI prompt you can use to check your medication list:

"Have any of the following drugs [drug names here] been found to cause drug-induced autoimmunity? Do any of these drugs contain heavy metals, including aluminum, or additives, fillers, or excipients that are linked to chronic inflammation?"

This prompt should give you some idea of whether or not drug-induced autoimmunity could be part of the problem. This is not a recommendation to stop any medication, but rather it should serve as something to discuss with your practitioner.

VACCINES AND AUTOIMMUNITY

There is little controversy around drug-induced autoimmunity. Vaccines are another story, and one I must be careful in writing about. I cannot share everything I think about this topic in a book that will be sold on major platforms. I trust you understand why.

What I can say is this. Vaccines, like all medical interventions, carry both potential benefits and potential risks. The adjuvants used in vaccines are designed to stimulate the immune system. In a person with a low toxic burden and strong repair capacity, that stimulus may be well-tolerated. However, for a person who is already overloaded, it may be the straw that breaks the camel's back.

This is the concept of toxicant-induced loss of tolerance. As the toxic burden rises, the immune system can lose its ability to distinguish what to attack from what to leave alone.[32] This includes tolerance to foods, chemicals, environmental allergens, and sometimes our own tissues.

Mark's Story: Occult Vasculitis and Vertigo

Mark came to see me for symptoms that started shortly after receiving a dose of one of the COVID-19 vaccines. He blamed the vaccine for his new health issues. He had been a successful tech-company founder who had been enjoying his retirement with his wife and family, including numerous grandchildren. After the COVID-19 vaccine, he developed severe vertigo and episodes of loss of consciousness. He worried he would not be well enough to be present for his family. A local doctor diagnosed him with low thyroid hormone and prescribed large doses of thyroid medication. He started losing weight rapidly.

When he came to see me, we ran comprehensive testing. His thyroid hormone levels were actually high, not low. He was depleted in multiple minerals and B vitamins. We corrected his thyroid dose and started a customized supplement protocol. He began gaining weight, his blood pressure normalized, and his vertigo stopped. His kidney function later showed signs of strain, and we continue to monitor it.

Mark had been a healthy, vibrant man before. There was no doubt in his mind that it was the COVID-19 vaccine that ruined his health.

I could fill a book with case studies and testimonies like Mark's.

WHAT THIS MEANS FOR YOU

"I cannot teach anybody anything; I can only make them think."

—Socrates

If you have autoimmunity, I encourage you to be cautious about what medical treatments and interventions you accept. Many of them are linked to autoimmunity. Consider your current level of repair deficit. Consider whether your toxic burden is already high. Have an honest conversation with a practitioner who understands these dynamics and is willing to engage in genuine risk-benefit analysis, rather than one-size-fits-all recommendations.

I have prepared a detailed article on Vaccines and Autoimmunity that contains everything I cannot say here. It includes the research, the mechanisms, the clinical observations, and the resources that have shaped my thinking. It also includes detailed case studies from my practice. You can review the evidence yourself and draw your own conclusions.

You'll find it in the companion resources at stillmanmd.com/autoimmunity.

Next, we need to talk about how our buildings and indoor lifestyles can drive autoimmunity.

SICK BUILDING SYNDROME AND AUTOIMMUNITY

Sick buildings make people sick. What do I mean by sick buildings? And how do they make people sick?

Most people spend over 90 percent of their time indoors. There are many causes of sick building syndrome, including electrosmog, indoor air pollution, and artificial light.

Here are the key screening questions I ask to detect sick building syndrome:

- Do your symptoms clearly improve when you are away from the building for several days? Yes / No
- Did an illness arise shortly after moving into a new home or apartment, or after taking a new job? Yes / No
- Do you often notice musty, moldy, or chemical odors in the building? Yes / No
- Is anyone else in the building sick? Yes / No
- Do you feel like no matter what you do, you never feel better? Yes / No
- Are you a "mystery" to doctors, friends, and families? Yes / No
- Do you feel "stuck" even though you have great doctors who understand root-cause medicine? Yes / No

If you answered yes to any of the above, then I encourage you to check out "What's in Your Home That's Confusing Your Immune System?" and "Healthy Homes for Healthy Families" in the companion resources at stillmanmd.com/autoimmunity.

EMOTIONS AND AUTOIMMUNITY

Our immune system truly begins in our brain and is intricately connected to our hearts. Doctors once thought autoimmunity was a matter of immune confusion and a purely biochemical event. Recent research has shown strong associations between our emotions and autoimmunity.[33] Many patients with autoimmunity are carrying burdens they may not even recognize as drivers of their disease.

Learn more about how emotions and relationships can drive autoimmunity in the companion resource, "Healing the Wounded Heart," at stillmanmd.com/autoimmunity.

AVOIDING THE HAZARDS OF MODERN LIFE

If you found this chapter discouraging or alarming, I want to offer you hope. Life is richer, fuller, and more joyful without these hazards. Many of them are distractions from our hopes and dreams. Who will look back at their life and think, "I wish I had spent more time on my cell phone?" My experience taking care of patients in their final days and hours is that what they want most is more quality time with their family. Creating the healthy and meaningful relationships that matter most to us starts with creating healthy environments and lifestyles, so our bodies are healthy. That is what this chapter is truly about.

Most of our patients are pleased with their results, even if they do not tackle all the hazards in this chapter. I hope you will be so encouraged by the results you see that you will continue on until you have created the healthiest life possible.

YOUR NEXT STEP

Start the 14-Day Detox when you are ready. If you need a reminder of the five swaps, turn back to the beginning of this chapter or download the checklist from the companion resources at stillmanmd.com/autoimmunity.

Take the Repair Deficit Survey every two weeks at stillmanmd.com/autoimmunity. As you eliminate hazards, watch how your score changes. Healing is not linear. Some symptoms may worsen before they improve, and scores sometimes rise before they fall. This is normal. Your score over time tells you whether you are heading in the right direction.

There is so much more for me to share with you about hazards. You can find them in the companion resources at stillmanmd.com/autoimmunity.

You can submit questions for our Q&A shows at stillmanmd.com/autoimmunity.

You now know what to add to your life and what to remove. But every person's situation is unique. How do you know which specific imbalances are driving your repair deficit? How do you know what to prioritize? Now, we turn to the diagnostics we rely on in our practice.

COMPANION RESOURCES FOR CHAPTER 4

The companion resources at stillmanmd.com/autoimmunity bring together everything you need to identify and eliminate hazards. You will find:

- Resources for Personal Care Products, Clothing, Kitchen Gear, and More
- What's in Your Home That's Confusing Your Immune System?
- Healthy Homes for Healthy Families
- Vaccines and Autoimmunity

You can submit questions about hazards for our Q&A shows at stillmanmd.com/autoimmunity.

CHAPTER 5

Diagnostics

"Listen to the patient. He is telling you the diagnosis."

—William Osler, MD

How do we diagnose autoimmunity?

We see over a dozen different diagnoses in our practice each year. The most common are:

- Chronic fatigue syndrome
- Fibromyalgia
- Hashimoto's thyroiditis
- Graves' disease
- Rheumatoid arthritis
- Multiple sclerosis
- Granuloma annulare
- Myasthenia gravis
- Psoriasis
- Vitiligo
- Microscopic or lymphocytic colitis
- Aplastic anemia

- Crohn's disease
- Ulcerative colitis
- Lichen sclerosus
- Polymyalgia rheumatica

What do these seemingly different diseases have to do with one another? They are all driven by a repair deficit.

The diagnosis tells you what to call your condition. It doesn't tell you why you have it. Repair deficit is the process behind every autoimmune disease. The diagnosis is a label. The repair deficit is the problem.

I focus on the process rather than the label. One patient gets Sjogren's, another gets chronic fatigue syndrome, and another gets Crohn's disease. The diseases have different names, but the process is the same. Some patients have a formal diagnosis. Some have signs and symptoms, but no clear diagnosis. Regardless of diagnosis, the process and framework we follow are the same. We do personalize them on a case-by-case basis, but the majority of what we do is standardized (otherwise writing this book would have been impossible).

I chose the stories of John, Meredith, and Emily for Chapter 2 to illustrate this point. John had no formal diagnosis of autoimmunity. Meredith had one that is extremely common—chronic fatigue syndrome—but that has no test or blood markers to base the diagnosis on. There is no effective pharmaceutical treatment for chronic fatigue syndrome. Emily's diagnosis—myasthenia gravis—is well-defined by signs, symptoms, and strict diagnostic criteria. There are drugs and one surgical procedure to treat myasthenia. These stories range from "mystery illness" with no known treatment (John) to a vague diagnosis with no clear treatment (Meredith) to a well-defined diagnosis with clear treatment paths and protocols (Emily).

What mattered was not the diagnostic label, but the process and framework we used to restore health.

The diagnosis does not matter as much as you might think. That being said, the diagnosis is still useful. It is worth taking the time to diagnose autoimmune diseases, and that is what this chapter is about.

Diagnosing autoimmune diseases in the conventional sense means running blood tests for auto-antibodies specific to those diseases. It means obtaining biopsies of affected organs and examining them under a microscope. There are scoring questionnaires for diseases that have no blood markers.

If your blood tests or biopsies are negative, and you don't score enough points on your diagnostic questionnaires, most doctors conclude you do not have an autoimmune disease. Patients are left wondering what is wrong with them. If they wait long enough, many will develop positive blood tests or biopsies for autoimmunity. They will eventually score enough points to meet the criteria for an autoimmune disease.

I have always felt that waiting for a diagnosis is playing to lose. Imagine you are playing a team sport. Would you let the other team score points while you sit on your hands, only to start playing when the opposing team has reached a certain number of points?

One of the patterns I noticed in our practice, and that prompted me to write this book, was the similarity between the histories of different patients in our practice. Three diagnoses were most common and almost always preceded a full-blown autoimmune disease: irritable bowel syndrome, fibromyalgia, and chronic fatigue syndrome. Virtually all our autoimmune patients fit the criteria for one or more of these diseases. The literature bears this out. Patients with irritable bowel syndrome are 68 percent more likely to develop autoimmune bowel disease (inflammatory bowel disease) than those without.[34] Twenty percent of patients with multiple sclerosis meet the criteria for irritable bowel syndrome, which is twice the rate of those without multiple sclerosis.[35] Patients with fibromyalgia are around four to five times more likely to be diagnosed with autoimmune rheumatic diseases like rheumatoid arthritis or lupus in the following years than those without fibromyalgia.[36] Many patients with chronic fatigue syndrome show evidence of autoimmune activity, and autoimmune diseases such as Hashimoto's thyroiditis, psoriasis, and rheumatoid arthritis appear more frequently in patients with chronic fatigue syndrome than in the general population.[37] I stopped worrying about the diagnosis when it became apparent that common root causes were driving these diseases.

When I started in private practice, I applied our framework to all our patients, regardless of diagnosis. It worked well for patients regardless of their diagnosis. Individual results varied widely, for many reasons, but overall, patients were overwhelmingly happy with their results.

Today, many patients come to us because they have already adopted many of the essentials and mitigated many of the hazards covered in this book, and yet they have not recovered their health. They feel like they have tried everything. They know the answer must be in diagnostics and therapeutics.

Diagnostics are essential to our success. This chapter will show you what we test, why it matters, and how to use testing to accelerate your results.

WHAT ACTUALLY DRIVES RESULTS

Testing doesn't directly create results. Testing quantifies repair deficit and root causes like nutritional deficiencies, toxins, and infections. We use this data to make better decisions. I see many patients failing to get great results, despite an abundance (and sometimes an over-abundance) of lab testing. The data we gather is only as good as the treatment plan it allows us to personalize based on it. Results come when we pay down the repair deficit. You don't pay this down in one day or with one action. You pay it down with many small acts, done over time.

I ask patients whenever they report a major improvement in their health, "What gets the credit?" Rarely do they give 50 percent or more credit to one thing. They almost always credit a combination of diet and lifestyle changes, along with supplements and sometimes drugs. Don't take my word for it. Listen to podcasts with people like Amy, Meredith, Emily, Ashlee, and Jim, and hear what they have to say about what worked, and sometimes what didn't.

Testing helps us personalize and optimize. It helps us get better results faster. But it is no substitute for the Principles, Essentials, and Hazards. I've seen patients ignore those three and spend all their time and money on Diagnostics and Therapeutics, only to get worse results than people who just took the time optimizing their Principles, Essentials, and Hazards.

We start with a simple scoring tool: the Repair Deficit Survey.

YOUR STARTING POINT: THE REPAIR DEFICIT SURVEY

This survey is how we quantify and track repair deficit in our patients. You can take it online at stillmanmd.com/autoimmunity.

There are seven questions covering different symptom "domains."

SCORING SEVERITY

- Zero means never or not at all.
- One means mild—present occasionally, noticeable effect on comfort or function.
- Two means moderate—present regularly, noticeable effect on comfort or function.
- Three means marked—frequent, clearly limits activities or performance.
- Four means severe—constant or nearly constant, disabling or very distressing.

Rate the following seven domains on this zero-to-four scale.

THE SEVEN DOMAINS

- **Domain 1:** Fatigue, sleepiness, lack of drive, low motivation, or low mood.
- **Domain 2:** Weight loss, weight gain, appetite control, or water retention.
- **Domain 3:** Pain, including headaches, joint pain, back pain, and neck pain.
- **Domain 4:** Brain fog, memory issues, poor comprehension, poor concentration, or confusion.
- **Domain 5:** Chest pain, shortness of breath, exercise intolerance, poor recovery from exercise, anxiety, or feelings of overwhelm.
- **Domain 6:** Rashes, acne, skin dryness, hair loss, excessive sweating, or lack of ability to sweat.
- **Domain 7:** Indigestion, constipation, diarrhea, bloating, or other digestive symptoms.

Your total score (maximum twenty-eight) gives you a baseline. Track it every two weeks to measure your progress. Don't be discouraged if it gets worse before it gets better—that is typical. Patients who only get better are, in fact, the exception rather than the rule.

This survey is our most important tracking tool. It helps us ensure our patients are making progress.

If you want printable versions of the Repair Deficit Survey, you will find them at stillmanmd.com/autoimmunity.

Now let's look at how laboratory testing can accelerate your progress.

LANA'S STORY: RAPIDLY REVERSING REPAIR DEFICIT

Lana came to us struggling with chronic fatigue syndrome, fibromyalgia, and irritable bowel syndrome. She could barely work. Eight-hour days had become two hours, if she was lucky. She was exhausted, in pain, and constantly bloated. She stopped calling friends and family out of fear that she would forget a name or an important fact about them. She stopped going out because she was just too exhausted. She had no energy for hobbies, vacations, or exercise. She had a loving and supportive husband, wonderful friends, and a beautiful home, but between her fatigue, brain fog, and pain, she was missing out on the wonderful life that she had spent years building.

Her Repair Deficit Survey score reflected her misery. Every domain was moderate to severe. Her exact score was 24, with fatigue, brain fog, pain, and digestive issues being the most severe.

We ran comprehensive labs. Here's what we found.

- Her copper was 122 mcg/dL, with optimal being less than 100 mcg/dL.
- Her zinc was 88 mcg/dL, with optimal being 105–120 mcg/dL.
- Her iron saturation was 45 percent, with optimal being 25–35 percent.
- Her ferritin was 199, with optimal being less than 150 ng/ml.
- Her hair tissue test showed low levels of minerals, which is what we expect in patients who feel exhausted.

Her labs were only mildly abnormal. Her symptoms, however, were severe. A patient's symptoms are often much, much more severe than their labs would suggest. Likewise, we often find that patients with few symptoms have many signs of repair deficit on lab testing.

We started personalized supplements targeting her imbalances, along with the diet and lifestyle changes from Chapters 3 and 4.

Three months later, Lana reported 95 percent improvement in fatigue, brain fog, and gut issues.

Her Repair Deficit Survey score dropped into the single digits. She was back to working full days. Her pain disappeared. Her bloating resolved.

I usually recommend testing labs again at three-month intervals, but we never did for Lana. I share this story with you to show how simple this approach can be. Lana's severe symptoms dramatically improved in just a few months thanks to the framework. We were guided by only a few lab abnormalities in a panel consisting of hundreds of markers.

Lana's elevated copper and iron, and low zinc, were the result of years of accumulated repair deficit. The initial labs helped us personalize her supplement protocol. The survey told us she was moving in the right direction.

What lab tests do we routinely run in our practice? There is a panel I have designed after years of testing to cover the most important biomarkers for patients with autoimmunity.

THE REPAIR DEFICIT PANEL: FOURTEEN MARKERS THAT PREDICT YOUR FUTURE

"What gets measured gets managed."

—Peter Drucker

After reviewing thousands of labs over more than twelve years of practice, I've chosen fourteen blood markers that consistently predict repair deficit. These are not all of the markers I rely on. There is much more information about lab testing at stillmanmd.com/autoimmunity. These fourteen markers tell us how severe your repair deficit is and what needs attention most urgently. We call them "The Repair Deficit Panel."

These fourteen markers are the bottom line of your body's repair bank account. They show whether you are in the red or the black. They tell us whether you're gaining ground or falling behind. When these numbers move toward optimal, the repair deficit is resolving.

The Repair Deficit Panel includes the following markers, for which I have also included what I consider "optimal" ranges.

- Anti-Nuclear Antibody (ANA) detects autoimmunity. When positive, mortality risk increases by over fourfold.[38] Optimal is negative (undetectable).

- Albumin reflects nutritional status and liver function. Low levels predict death and disability. Optimal is 4.5–5.3 g/dL.
- Bilirubin shows how well you eliminate toxins via bile. High levels can indicate bile flow obstruction. Optimal is less than 1.0 mg/dL.
- Cardiac CRP measures inflammation. It is the single best predictor we have of life expectancy. Optimal is less than 1.0 mg/L.
- Ferritin is an iron storage protein. For every one-hundred-point rise above two hundred, mortality increases 10 percent. Optimal is less than 150 ng/mL.
- An Iron Panel includes serum iron, TIBC, and transferrin saturation. We care about transferrin saturation. High transferrin saturation indicates iron overload. Optimal transferrin saturation is 25–35 percent.
- Magnesium is essential for energy generation, brain and nerve function, and blood flow. Deficiency is extremely common, particularly in autoimmunity. Optimal is 2.1–2.4 mg/dL.
- Copper is toxic in excess and essential in the right amounts. Mortality starts to rise quickly with blood levels above 103.[39] Optimal is 80–100 mcg/dL.
- Zinc is critical for immune function. Most people are deficient. The top quartile (greater than 96 mcg/dL) has significantly better outcomes. Optimal is 105–120 mcg/dL.
- Homocysteine reflects methylation and detoxification capacity. It also indicates toxic burden. Optimal is less than 9 μmol/L.
- Urinary pH (first morning void) reflects mineral reserves and metabolic health. Optimal is around 7.0.

- Free T3 is the active thyroid hormone. Higher levels predict better outcomes and longer life.[40] Optimal is greater than 3.4 pg/mL.
- Hemoglobin A1C is an average of blood glucose over three months. A sweet spot exists. Too low or too high both increase mortality. Optimal is 5.2–5.6 percent.
- Fibrinogen is a clotting protein and marker of inflammation. Lower is better. Optimal is less than 285 mg/dL.

These markers tell us where you are on the spectrum from optimal health to severe repair deficit. The worse they look, the more urgently we need to intervene. The better they look, the closer you are to resolving the repair deficit.

We trend these markers over time because a repair deficit doesn't resolve overnight. It takes years to develop. It takes months or years to reverse. Tracking these markers shows us we're heading in the right direction and helps us adjust protocols as we go.

Now let's see how tracking specific abnormal markers can guide treatment decisions.

DAVID'S STORY: METALS, FATIGUE, AND GUT DYSFUNCTION

David came to us with fatigue, brain fog, and gut issues. He had seen many doctors, but was still struggling. He was a successful entrepreneur at the height of his career. He was frustrated that his medical issues were interfering with his ability to provide for his family and secure their future. He wanted to be able to travel, pursue his career, and enjoy his life with his family.

His labs revealed a severe repair deficit.

David's initial labs from September 2020 and January 2021 showed the following:

- Ferritin was 355 ng/mL. Optimal is less than 150 ng/mL.
- Transferrin saturation was 47 percent. Optimal is 25 to 35 percent.
- Zinc was 72 mcg/dL. Optimal is 105 to 120 mcg/dL.
- Mercury was 73.0 nmol/L. Normal is less than 25.0 nmol/L. Optimal is effectively zero, although that is hard to reach in the modern world.

David's main problem was iron overload combined with severe mercury toxicity. His mercury was nearly three times the upper limit of normal. The ferritin of 355 ng/mL was highly concerning, given its strong association with shorter life and reduced quality of life. Both iron and mercury were displacing zinc and crippling his ability to repair.

He started to donate blood to reduce his iron overload. We also started personalized mineral supplementation.

Four months later, in September 2022, he had made significant improvement. His energy levels had risen. His thinking was clearer. He felt like a new man.

But his labs did not all "normalize" overnight. Some numbers moved in the right direction. Others looked worse on paper before they improved.

This is a reality that many patients and practitioners fail to appreciate. You have to trend labs to catch new abnormalities and to confirm that old abnormalities have finally normalized. You have to accept that some results will look worse before they get better.

Patients operating without practitioner guidance are likely to get turned around. They say things like "I took zinc, but my zinc fell, what happened?" or "I am doing everything right, but my homocysteine rose, what is going on?" This is a process. Healing does not happen overnight. Healing is not linear. Labs fluctuate, which is why trending them is so important.

David's labs in September 2022, one year after his first round of testing, showed the following:

- Zinc had risen to 94 mcg/dL. This was better than 72, but still short of the optimal 105 to 120 mcg/dL.
- Copper had dropped to 58 mcg/dL. It had been 87 before, which was in the ideal range of 80 to 100 mcg/dL. Copper looks worse, but in the context of high ferritin and mercury, we expected copper to shift as we moved metals and minerals.
- Iron had risen to 181 mcg/dL. This looks worse than his first iron value of 132.
- Ferritin had dropped to 103 ng/mL, a major improvement from 355 and now well under the 150 ng/mL threshold.
- Transferrin saturation had risen to 76 percent. This looks much worse than his previous 47 percent, given that the optimal is 25–35 percent.

In his second round of lab testing:

- Ferritin looked clearly better.
- Zinc looked somewhat better.
- Iron and transferrin saturation looked worse.
- Copper looked worse.

His ferritin dropped after he donated blood, which is exactly what we expect. His iron and transferrin saturation rose, which often happens as stored iron is mobilized. His zinc rose, while his copper fell.

This did not surprise me. We often see shifts like this, from better to worse, before we see labs enter the optimal range.

We did not panic. We did not run in the opposite direction. Reviewing thousands of these panels has taught me that sometimes numbers go up before they go down. We stuck to the framework. We kept doing what we know works, and David continued to improve. Based on his clinical improvement—more energy, less brain fog, better gut function—I knew we were headed in the right direction.

Nearly three years after his first round of labs, in August 2024, his results finally lined up with what we had been seeing clinically since 2022.

- Zinc had dropped slightly from 94 mcg/dL to 87 mcg/dL, still short of the 105 to 120 mcg/dL target but stable.
- Copper had risen from 58 mcg/dL to 80 mcg/dL, now in the acceptable range below 100 mcg/dL.
- Iron had dropped from 181 mcg/dL to 83 mcg/dL.
- Ferritin was essentially unchanged at 109 ng/mL, still under 150 ng/mL.
- Transferrin saturation had dropped from 76 percent to 27 percent. This is optimal.

Here is a table of his full lab progression for those who prefer to see the numbers side-by-side:

David's Lab Progression Table

Marker	Optimal Range	Initial (Sept. 2020/Jan. 2021)	Sept. 2022	Aug. 2024
Ferritin	Less than 150 ng/mL	355 ng/mL	103 ng/mL	109 ng/mL
Transferrin Saturation	25 to 35 percent	47 percent	76 percent	27 percent
Zinc	105 to 120 mcg/dL	72 mcg/dL	94 mcg/dL	87 mcg/dL
Mercury	Less than 25.0 nmol/L	73.0 nmol/L	Not tested	Not tested
Copper	80 to 100 mcg/dL	87 mcg/dL	58 mcg/dL	80 mcg/dL
Iron	Less than 150 mcg/dL	132 mcg/dL	181 mcg/dL	83 mcg/dL

David had made substantial progress, but his labs were still not optimal even after two years. This is not uncommon, and I mention it specifically to prepare patients for the reality that this can be a long process. Clinically, his symptoms resolved. Energy returned. Brain fog lifted. Gut issues disappeared.

Tracking these specific abnormal markers over time was critical. The numbers didn't improve linearly. They fluctuated as his body rebalanced. Ferritin came down quickly, but transferrin saturation increased before dropping into the optimal range. Iron actually rose, despite his donating blood, and only fell later on. Zinc rose and then fell as minerals redistributed.

David made rapid progress over his first year and continued to make progress in subsequent years. This was based on multiple rounds of blood work within this time frame. I share his story to make the point that labs must be repeated so we can personalize treatment.

Most patients only order annual labs. Do you change the oil

in your car once a year? Do you check your bank balance once a year? Do you check on your parents, kids, or grandparents once a year?

Of course not. You check in on these things periodically to make sure everything and everyone is okay.

David's case is a great example of how radically labs can change, and sometimes in ways that patients and practitioners do not expect and that even seem paradoxical.

For best results (fastest, most durable, and most significant), we recommend testing every quarter, and no less than every four months. We may extend this to every six months on a case-by-case basis.

David had been making withdrawals from his body's repair bank account that he didn't know about. Iron and mercury had poisoned him slowly. Testing revealed what years of symptoms couldn't explain. Once we knew what the problem was, we could solve it.

But blood work alone doesn't tell the whole story. The Repair Deficit Panel includes the most important blood labs that I order on a daily basis. But hair mineral and metal levels are a cornerstone of our practice, as we will discuss next.

COMPANION RESOURCES FOR BLOOD TESTING

If you're curious to learn more about blood testing, you'll find more companion resources on this topic at stillmanmd.com/autoimmunity. I cover the Repair Deficit Panel in more detail in "Why Your Labs Are 'Normal' When You Feel Terrible." You'll get more information on the Comprehensive Wellness Panel, which includes the Repair Deficit Panel, and I share my own personal lab testing results so you can see what is possible.

HAIR TISSUE MINERAL ANALYSIS: THE TEST MOST DOCTORS MISS

"You can trace every sickness, every disease, and every ailment to a mineral deficiency."

—Linus Pauling

If you're working with a practitioner and can only add one test beyond basic bloodwork, this is my favorite.

Hair Tissue Mineral Analysis (HTMA) measures mineral and metal levels in your hair. You cut a small sample from the back of your head, mail it to the lab, and get results in a few weeks.

Blood testing shows you a snapshot. It could be a high or a low point. Hair testing is your running average over months and years. It reveals the withdrawals your body has been making over long periods of time. It is arguably our best test for visualizing the repair deficit over time.

HTMA reveals heavy metal elimination. When toxic metals like mercury, lead, aluminum, or cadmium appear in hair testing, it often means your body is finally eliminating them. Blood testing often misses this entirely. I include detailed case studies in the companion resources online to prove this point.

The patterns we see in hair testing tell us exactly which minerals to supplement and in what amounts. I've seen this outperform one-size-fits-all approaches in case after case.

HTMA shows changes over time, without the noise of highs and lows we see in blood testing. As you saw in David's case, he donated blood, but his blood iron levels rose. This presents a paradox. Why would reducing the body's iron stores with blood donation result in rising blood levels of iron? There is a surprising amount of "noise" in blood labs. For most lab markers, a 20 percent variation from day to day is typical. For some markers, you will see swings of 100 percent or more.

Knowing this is critical for proper lab interpretation. Most practitioners do not understand these realities, which is why patients so often feel "terrible" when their labs are "normal." Much of this comes down to a variation in blood levels of hormones, nutrients, and other biomarkers.

Hair testing helps us cut out this noise. Hair mineral and metal levels are a running average over the life of the hair follicle. We track these changes because what patients need in month four may differ radically from what they need in month one. We adjust our supplement protocols quarterly based on HTMA for this reason.

Here is a story of the kind of progressions we see with HTMA in mineral and metal levels, and how life-changing this testing can be.

PHILIP'S STORY: POISONED BY MERCURY, COPPER, AND ALUMINUM

Philip came to us at age eighteen with Crohn's colitis. He was on immunosuppressive medications to control his disease, but his parents noticed major changes in his mood and behavior with these drugs. His parents were concerned about what these drugs might do to him long term. They wondered how they might affect his personality for the rest of his life. Unfortunately, most drugs are not studied for long enough to rule out these concerns. We discovered after decades of prescribing that inhaled steroids for asthma and allergies actually stunted growth in patients by a few inches. What else did it do to them? We may never know.

Philip's parents wanted their son to be healthy, not dependent upon drugs to keep a crippling disease at bay.

His initial testing revealed a severe repair deficit.

- Albumin was 3.6 g/dL. The optimal range is 4.5 to 5.3 g/dL.
- Serum copper was 181 mcg/dL. Optimal is less than 100 mcg/dL.
- Zinc was 53 mcg/dL. Optimal is 105 to 120 mcg/dL.
- Cardiac CRP was 129.93 mg/L. Optimal is less than 1.0 mg/L.

His hair testing told the rest of the story.

Copper in the hair was 2,500 mcg%, which is a normal level for the hair and is low compared to the level in his blood.

Lead, mercury, cadmium, and arsenic were all extremely low.

Aluminum was elevated at 1,490 mcg%. This was the only clearly elevated heavy metal on his first panel.

The albumin of 3.6 g/dL indicated malnutrition. The cardiac CRP of 129.93 mg/L showed extreme inflammation, more than one hundred times the acceptable level. The copper of 181 mcg/dL was partly responsible for this. The zinc of 53 mcg/dL was roughly half of what we consider optimal.

We started a personalized supplement protocol to balance his minerals, metals, and metabolism. He also remained on strong immunosuppressants from his gastroenterologist.

Five months later, we retested.

- Cardiac CRP was 0.34 mg/L. Optimal is less than 1.0 mg/L.
- Copper was 110 mcg/dL. Optimal is less than 100 mcg/dL.
- Zinc was 81 mcg/dL. Optimal is 105 to 120 mcg/dL.

His cardiac CRP had dropped from 129.93 to 0.34 mg/L. His copper had fallen from 181 to 110 mcg/dL. His zinc had risen from 53 to 81 mcg/dL.

On hair testing, copper was now 5,300 mcg% and aluminum was 2,880 mcg%. Copper in the hair had more than doubled, and aluminum had almost doubled, showing that his body was finally pushing these metals out.

Why did his hair copper and aluminum almost double, when he had done everything we recommended to reduce aluminum exposure, and his blood copper had dropped nearly in half?

This is the paradox of hair testing. We often find that what the body has too much of is actually low in the hair. What the body does not have enough of is often wasted in the hair. Patients with a significant repair deficit typically cannot eliminate the heavy metals they have accumulated, which are wreaking havoc on their bodies. I showed you Lana and David's blood iron studies earlier, but I didn't mention their hair iron levels were low. This is the rule, rather than the exception.

What is behind this paradoxical finding?

Imagine a city that has run out of money and resources. The trash trucks are not running. No trash is leaving the city. The wrong conclusion would be that an absence of trash trucks means an absence of trash. In 1968, New York Sanitation workers went on strike for nine days. Over 100,000 tons of trash piled up in the streets. New York City accumulated a 100,000 ton "trash removal deficit" over just nine days. Just because the trash trucks aren't running doesn't mean there is no trash in need of removal.

This is exactly how we look at a repair deficit. Imagine your body's detoxification services go on strike due to a lack of minerals, vitamins, sleep, sunlight, and more. The toxins pile up. The strike ends. Your body doesn't take out all that trash at once.

Your body takes that trash out starting at the top and working its way down.

The remarkable trend in our practice is that as we treat our patients to resolve their repair deficit, toxic metal levels tend to rise in their hair, rather than declining. Waves of heavy metals come out as the body regains the energy and nutrients necessary to finally eliminate them.

Four months later, we tested Philip again. His tests had changed significantly yet again.

Hair testing showed copper had dropped to 1,000 mcg%. This was lower than his initial hair copper level, indicating he had eliminated excess copper from his body.

Aluminum had dropped to 620 mcg%. His body was no longer eliminating it.

However, mercury had risen to 131 mcg%.

As copper cleared, Philip's body mobilized aluminum. As aluminum cleared, his body began mobilizing mercury. The body did not try to eliminate all these toxins at once.

In his most recent hair test, his mercury has risen further to 158 mcg%. These are levels that often correlate with elevated mercury in the blood. David, in our earlier story, had lower levels of hair mercury than Philip, and his blood mercury levels were markedly elevated. The body tends to hide heavy metals. When even modest elevations are found in hair, it consistently indicates that significant detoxification is underway.

Philip's Hair Testing Results Over Time

Metal	Test 1	Test 2	Test 3	Test 4
Copper	2,500	5,300	1,000	1,300
Aluminum	1,490	2,880	620	1,050
Mercury	27	44	131	158

All values in mcg%

What This Means

The body doesn't eliminate all of its heavy metals in a few months. It may have been storing them for years. This is why we see copper, then aluminum, and then mercury rising in Philip's hair. His body is taking the trash out one truck at a time.

This is why quarterly HTMA testing is so valuable. Philip's healing progressed in waves. We may see more copper, aluminum, mercury, or other heavy metals in future tests. The body can store enormous quantities of heavy metals in vital organs and bones that are difficult to measure and even more difficult to eliminate.

Had we tested annually instead of quarterly, we would have missed each transition entirely. We wouldn't have known how to adjust his protocols at each phase.

Had we done blood work alone without HTMA, we would never have seen the aluminum or mercury eliminations. These metals don't show reliably in blood testing, even if the body has a significant burden of them.

Quarterly HTMA plus blood work catches these critical transitions as your biochemistry changes. This is a cornerstone of our approach.

What you need in month one differs from month four, which differs from month eight, which differs from month twelve. This is a process. We have to adjust our protocols based on data, ideally collected quarterly.

THE GOOD, BETTER, BEST APPROACH TO LAB TESTING

Now that you understand what we test and why, let's talk about testing based on your resources and goals.

Good means annual Repair Deficit Panel testing. You might consider our entire Comprehensive Wellness Panel, which you can learn more about at stillmanmd.com/autoimmunity. I strongly urge you to work with a clinician to order and interpret lab testing.

Better means an annual Repair Deficit Panel and quarterly follow-up. We retest any abnormal markers quarterly until patients reach optimal ranges. Quarterly follow-up on these specific markers is ideal to track progress and confirm that what we are doing is working.

Best means at least an annual HTMA and our Comprehensive Wellness Panel (which includes the Repair Deficit Panel, plus many more markers), with quarterly retesting of hair and blood. We repeat abnormal tests as often as every six to twelve weeks. Testing every quarter allows for greater precision, which leads to faster results, more consistently.

Don't feel like you "need" best. Most of our patients start with "best," but once they reach their goals, we only check labs once yearly. Annual labs make sense for patients who feel and function well, and have optimal labs or nearly optimal labs.

If you're curious to see my labs and to learn why I believe so strongly in this approach, check out the companion resources at stillmanmd.com/autoimmunity. I share the results of years of lab testing I have done on myself. They show you what is possible and what to expect.

ALLERGY AND IMMUNE RESPONSE TESTING

"What is food to one man may be fierce poison to others."

—Lucretius

Food or environmental triggers often drive autoimmunity. When patients eliminate their allergic triggers, symptoms can improve dramatically, sometimes within hours.

The challenge is identifying what you're reacting to. Elimination diets work but require strict discipline. Testing can accelerate the process.

As I explained in Chapter 3 with Mary's story, food allergy testing identified corn as her trigger, leading to 90 percent improvement in her crippling abdominal pain. Cases like Mary's demonstrate why we recommend allergy testing for patients with autoimmunity.

Why do some patients develop allergies or autoimmunity associated with foods, food additives, or environmental allergens? As a repair deficit accumulates, the immune system loses control over what it attacks. Imagine a police force in a major city. How do they tell the difference between dangerous, violent criminals, nonviolent criminals, their friends and family, and innocent bystanders? How do they tell the difference between undercover police and criminals, or corrupt police and honest police?

There are many ways we distinguish friends from foes. Police wear uniforms. Criminals often have tattoos, gear, colors, or clothing specific to a gang. If you gather evidence, you can sort through it and figure out who is guilty and who is innocent. Now imagine you have a city that has few, if any, resources, and a badly compromised justice system. Imagine judges and police are being bribed to frame innocent people and let the guilty go. This is what a body in a state of repair deficit is like. The system that is supposed to deliver justice (in our process, this would be balancing nutrients, eliminating toxins and stress, and destroying pathogens) is broken.

What happens when we lose this tolerance? The immune system attacks everything from pollen to gluten to cow's milk protein, thinking these are dangerous pathogens or toxins that threaten your life. This creates tissue damage, as your cells and tissues are caught in the crossfire of an immune system trying to attack something that is as harmless as food. We can regain this tolerance, but it takes time. It takes effort. It takes consistency.

We use specialized immune testing that looks beyond standard allergy panels. Many patients have immune reactions that don't show up on typical allergy tests.

When allergy testing is positive, it can solve cases that seem hopeless. On the other hand, many patients see excellent results without allergy testing. It is not necessary for great results.

Get our most up-to-date recommendations on allergy testing in the companion resources at stillmanmd.com/autoimmunity.

YOUR NEXT STEP

You have learned what we test, why it matters, and how to approach testing based on your resources. You have seen through real cases how testing helps us implement the framework more precisely.

Testing is your roadmap. The Repair Deficit Survey shows

you where you are every two weeks. Lab testing helps you personalize protocols and verify you are heading in the right direction.

Your next step is to create a clear plan for lab testing. To make that easier, I created a short companion guide called "Autoimmune Lab Testing Secrets: How to Stop Wasting Time and Money on Useless Labs." In it, I show you which labs to prioritize, which ones to skip, and how to order testing in a way that protects your time, your budget, and your peace of mind.

You'll find it, along with all of the companion resources, at stillmanmd.com/autoimmunity.

Testing alone does not heal you. Diagnostics point the way, but therapeutics get you there. Chapter 6 is where testing turns into treatment.

COMPANION RESOURCES FOR CHAPTER 5

The Chapter 5 companion resources at stillmanmd.com/autoimmunity bring together everything you need to test and track your progress. You will find:

- The Repair Deficit Survey in printable form
- Technical guides for the Repair Deficit Panel and Comprehensive Wellness Panel
- Our Metals, Minerals, and Autoimmunity guide for understanding hair testing
- Guides for allergy testing, mold testing, organic acids, and Lyme
- "Autoimmune Lab Testing Secrets: How to Stop Wasting Time and Money on Useless Labs"
- Complete case studies with full lab progressions

You can submit questions about testing for our Q&A shows at stillmanmd.com/autoimmunity.

CHAPTER 6

Therapeutics

"The greatest medicine of all is teaching people how not to need it."

—Hippocrates

I became a doctor to help people feel, look, and perform at their best. It is my obsession. My wife can tell you I struggle to take time off from learning, thinking, and doing this work. The Essentials are essential, and you must avoid the Hazards that cause autoimmunity, but they do not require my medical degree or license to learn and implement. Therapeutics are where I spend 90 percent of my time in my daily practice. Diagnostics inform our therapeutics, and these two things together are why people come to see us from all over the world.

This chapter shares the therapeutics that consistently deliver results in our practice.

I share these through a "Good, Better, Best" framework, similar to previous chapters. Good executed consistently over a long enough period of time often gets the same results as Best. The faster you move, the more expensive your results will tend to be. The foundational protocols I share here take many of our patients all the way to their goal. You can Climb the Therapeutic Tree to get better results faster. If Best is not available to you, don't lose hope. Most people don't need Best to feel great every day.

Results vary tremendously. Some patients do only a little of what is in this book and get great results. Others do everything and still struggle.

How do you know which approach you need? Look at your Repair Deficit Survey score and your lab testing results. The higher your scores and the more lab abnormalities you have, the more you may benefit from Better or Best. Start with Good. You can always add more later.

Before we talk about therapeutics, we need to talk about what we need to thrive in our modern world.

WHAT WE NEED TO THRIVE IN OUR MODERN WORLD

"If you want to understand the secrets of the universe, think in terms of energy, frequency, and vibration."

—NIKOLA TESLA

When I think about what we need to thrive, I break everything down into two categories. We need energy, and we need matter.

We are living in an exciting time for light and energy medicine. This is no longer science fiction. Light therapy is fast becoming a clinical reality that offers new hope to patients.

Energy is the light you live under and the electromagnetic forces of the universe around you. Matter is the minerals, vitamins, proteins, fats, carbohydrates, and water that constitute our physical bodies.

As we covered in earlier chapters, our environment has

changed drastically. Our soil is depleted.[41] Our food is processed. We spend most of our time indoors away from natural light. We are exposed to toxins and electromagnetic frequencies that did not exist a century ago. This is why therapeutics matter.

As we discussed in Chapter 3, our indoor lifestyles rob us of healing frequencies of light. Sunlight is approximately 42 percent infrared light. Your average fluorescent bulb or LED emits zero infrared. Our bodies work best in an environment that is rich in infrared and red light. Without it, they cannot produce energy efficiently. I look at light as a nutrient. Life needs the right light to grow properly as much as it needs vitamins and minerals.

We need an abundance of nutrients, from minerals to frequencies of sunlight, to compensate for the toxic burden of our environment. Without these nutrients and with an increasing burden of toxins, repair deficit first appears and then grows. To restore health, we must restore the energy and matter necessary for good health to emerge.

How do energy and matter interact within our bodies?

Light, sound, and other forms of energy program and tune the human body. When bright light wakes you up in the morning, or a warm ray of summer sun puts you to sleep for an afternoon nap, light is "programming" your body. This is happening every second of every day, whether you realize it or not. Whether you are intentional with the energies that your body receives or not, it is receiving them.

The matter of your body, from your vital organs to your skin to your brain, is organized and directed by these energies. You need the right minerals, vitamins, amino acids, carbohydrates, and fats at all times for optimal health. You need precise amounts, and these amounts may vary over time.

Why do I start with this basic division between energy and matter?

Because everything we can pick up and wield as a therapeutic tool falls into one of these two categories. Energy and matter interact with one another. You must optimize both for good health.

WHERE TO START

I start therapeutics in a stepwise fashion. I have two goals in mind. First, do not overwhelm the patient practically or physically. If I give a patient a plan that doesn't fit into their daily life, I may do more harm than good due to anxiety and frustration. If I give a patient a plan that overwhelms their body's ability to adapt and heal, we are just wasting time and money. We may even trigger intolerable healing or detoxification reactions that disrupt their life. Paradoxically, sometimes less is more. When you pick and choose therapeutics thoughtfully, better results often come from somewhere between five and ten products daily.

> *"The young physician starts life with twenty drugs for each disease, and the old physician ends life with one drug for twenty diseases."*
>
> —Sir William Osler, MD

I have ten products that I rely upon in daily practice. There are dozens more products I use regularly, but these ten form the core of our approach. We start with a handful of these and rotate the rest in six-week cycles. These cycles keep the pill burden low and avoid disruptive healing or detoxification reactions. Judging by our patient satisfaction (we are in the top 10 percent of medical practices), patients love this approach for its simplicity and efficacy.

"Make things as simple as possible, but no simpler."

—Albert Einstein

How do I divide our approach into Good, Better, and Best?

I will cover these ten therapeutics in the order in which we start them in our practice.

I look at the first five—light therapy, minerals and vitamins, vitamin D, vitamin C, and digestive enzymes—as the bedrock of our approach. I generally continue these indefinitely.

These first five are Good.

For Better, we add supplements like SOD B, fish oil, choline citrate, and additional magnesium as needed. We also add high-dose protocols for nutrients like vitamins C or D.

For Best, we add bioidentical hormones, repurposed drugs, and other advanced therapeutics. In our practice, we personalize doses of vitamins and minerals based on lab testing.

You do not need to reach Best to get great results. Many of our most successful patients stay with Good, combined with the Essentials from Chapter 3 and the Hazards work from Chapter 4.

In many respects, your choice of Good, Better, or Best is not what matters most. Why do Chapters 3 and 4 precede Chapter 6? Because proper daily habits are essential for good health. Therapeutics without daily execution of the Essentials and regular avoidance of Hazards is like building a house on a cracked and crumbling foundation. You might build it well, and you might build it fast, but it is doomed to fall.

Good often trumps Best when patients take the Essentials and Hazards seriously. I have seen many wealthy, successful people fail to recover their health because they were too busy (distracted might be a better term) to execute them consistently. Money doesn't buy health.

The choice is yours. Start with Good. Add Better if needed. Choose Best if you can.

A NOTE ON PROTOCOLS

In this chapter, I am showing you what we do in our practice and why it works. I am describing our clinical approach, including the supplements we use, the order we use them in, and the results we see with patients under medical supervision.

What I am not doing is providing complete dosing protocols with every safety detail and nuance. There are two reasons for this.

First, complete protocols require individual medical supervision. What works for one patient may not work for another. Dosing must be adjusted based on response, side effects, and individual biochemistry.

Second, cramming every detail into this chapter would make it overwhelming and unusable. You would get lost in the weeds and miss the forest.

In the companion resources at stillmanmd.com/autoimmunity, you will find complete protocols with full dosing details, safety guardrails, side-effect management, and all the nuances we use in clinical practice. These are designed for you to review with your practitioner and only to implement under medical supervision. Note that I cannot endorse you using these without medical supervision.

If you have any questions, feel free to submit them at stillmanmd.com/autoimmunity.

Now, let us dive into therapeutics.

LIGHT THERAPY: OUR SAFEST AND MOST POWERFUL THERAPEUTIC

We start with light therapy because it is our safest and most powerful therapy. Sometimes, light therapy alone gets us the results we are looking for. Sometimes, light therapy gets us results that nothing else can. This is why we start light therapy with every patient who joins the practice.

The patients who get the best results in our practice use light therapy every single day. Light is one of the most powerful tools we have for creating wellness in our modern world. Learning to wield light is one of the most important things this book can teach you.

My friend, Kathleen Horstmeyer, has an incredible testimony as to the healing power of light. This is her story.

KATHLEEN'S STORY: HASHIMOTO'S, RUNAWAY INFLAMMATION, AND SEVERE SCARRING

Kathleen lives in Coeur d'Alene, Idaho. We met in 2022. She had a long history of Hashimoto's thyroiditis and severely elevated inflammatory markers on lab testing. Her high sensitivity C-reactive protein, our most well-validated marker for inflammation, had been in the "five" range for over two decades. This is squarely in the "high risk" range for future heart disease and other chronic diseases. She was struggling with her metabolism and energy. This was despite being a highly motivated, disciplined, and educated practitioner. She is a naturopathic doctor, respiratory therapist, and registered vascular specialist. Her husband is a doctor and a dentist. Kathleen was doing everything right. She had tried everything she could find.

Years before meeting me, she had been kicked in the abdomen by a horse and nearly died. The internal bleeding left her with a large rope-like scar that wrapped around roughly two-thirds of her lower abdomen and pelvis. She knew from her career teaching doctors how to read ultrasounds that scars can contribute to chronic disease later in life. She spent three years and hundreds of thousands of dollars on equipment to resolve the scar, with nothing to show for it. She was highly motivated to resolve it, but had run out of ways and means to do so.

Kathleen had tried many forms of light therapy over the course of her career. When I recommended a new light therapy product in my newsletter, she immediately ordered it. She started it not knowing what to expect. Within days, she noticed the scar felt different. At first, she dismissed this as her imagination. But the scar just kept getting smaller day by day.

After twelve days of light therapy, the scar had healed. She ran downstairs, shouting for joy to share the news with her husband. She called me and said, "Dr. Stillman, you're not going to believe this..."

I was floored. I had never seen anything like it.

We didn't stop with light therapy. We worked to improve her thyroid health, and she reduced her thyroid medication dose step by step, three separate times, under careful supervision. Her high sensitivity C-reactive protein dropped from the five range to 1.3 mg/L within about seven months, and a year later, it measured 1.0 mg/L.

Kathleen's case shows what can happen when you give cells the energy they need while supporting them with proper nutrition at the same time. Repairs that have been postponed for years can finally happen.

Kathleen and I recorded a podcast about her healing journey, including her experience with light therapy, in the companion resources at stillmanmd.com/autoimmunity.

HOW LIGHT THERAPY WORKS

Light tunes our mitochondria, the powerhouses of the cell, to operate at peak efficiency. Specific wavelengths of red and infrared light increase cellular energy production, improve blood flow, and enhance antioxidant defenses.[42] Light can also influence hormones, neurotransmitters, and peptides, which has profound effects on our health. This is why light therapy can affect so many different conditions. Light is a fundamental force of nature, and as such, it affects nature at the deepest levels possible.

Individual results vary, of course. Light therapy is not a magic bullet, but as a daily therapy inside the framework, it is one of the most powerful tools we have.

COMPANION RESOURCES FOR LIGHT THERAPY

To learn more about the light therapy that Kathleen used to heal, check out the companion resource "Healing with Light," at stillmanmd.com/autoimmunity. You will also find companion resources on UV light therapy, sauna therapy, and podcasts with Kathleen, Meredith, and others on the power of light therapy.

FROM LIGHT TO NUTRIENTS

Now that we have addressed light, we move to micronutrients. Micronutrients are present in tiny amounts, from microgram to gram quantities, in our daily diets. Our bodies need them for all critical physiologic processes, from movement to cellular repair. Without adequate vitamins and minerals, your cells have energy but nothing to build with. Without adequate light, your cells have materials but no energy to use them. You need both to resolve a repair deficit.

This is why the 14-Day Reset includes three ten-minute walks, a clear bedtime routine, and specific foods to include at each meal. You have already been optimizing the energy and matter of your body. This is why the 14-Day Detox eliminates products (matter) and reduces exposure to electrosmog and artificial light at night (energy).

The Essentials and Hazards are your foundation. Therapeutics build on them. This is why we don't even bother talking about Diagnostics and Therapeutics until more than halfway through the book.

Next, we will talk about supplements and products I use every day, both for myself and my family, and in our practice. For product details, see the "Supplements I Take Every Day" companion resource at stillmanmd.com/autoimmunity.

MINERALS AND VITAMINS: THE SPARK PLUGS OF LIFE

"The trace elements are more important in nutrition than are the vitamins, in the sense that they cannot be synthesized by living matter."

—Henry A. Schroeder, MD

The most important therapeutics we use in our practice are minerals and vitamins. These are the "spark plugs" of life, and modern people need them badly to resolve a repair deficit.

Unless you grow, hunt, or forage your own food without modern fertilizers, and then minimally process and prepare that food, your diet will be low in various minerals and vitamins, and contaminated with various toxins. We need vitamins and minerals to overcome the effects of toxins in our modern environment.

In our practice, we decide what supplements to use based on testing. If a patient has recent lab results, specifically HTMA and blood labs (like the Repair Deficit Panel), we will create a personalized supplement protocol for them. If they do not have recent lab results (recent means less than a month old), we use our high-quality multi-mineral/vitamin to support their mineral and vitamin levels. What this looks like in practice is that patients start with testing to enable personalized supplement protocols. We run testing quarterly and personalize their supplement protocols with each round of testing. When their labs are optimal and they've reached their goals, we have a discussion about whether or not to continue with personalized supplements and quarterly testing. Many of our patients continue to run lab testing every quarter indefinitely. Some decide to take a break and use our high-quality multi-mineral/vitamin to maintain optimal nutrient levels.

What vitamins and minerals do we use? That's a long story for a companion resource. Our framework includes every element of the periodic table and every vitamin so far discovered. Our personalized supplement protocols may include dozens of ingredients, carefully selected and dosed for each patient.

A word of caution about multi-vitamins and multi-minerals. Most "multis" are a waste of money. They use poor-quality ingredients and production methods that leave you with an inconsistent or even unsafe product. I spent years looking for a product I liked, and finally found one we now use in our practice. I based this decision on data from thousands of labs from hundreds of cases of autoimmune patients.

A few vitamins and minerals deserve dedicated entries here in the book. The first of these is vitamin D.

VITAMIN D

"A vitamin is something that makes you ill if you don't eat it."

—Albert Szent-Gyorgi

Vitamin D is technically a nutrient, but it functions as a hormone in the body. While we can absorb it from our food and make it within our skin from sunlight, modern people who rarely eat fish and spend little time outside are bound to be deficient in vitamin D.

Vitamin D is essential for immune function, bone health, mood regulation, and countless other processes. Low vitamin D is associated with increased risk of autoimmunity, cancer, heart disease, and depression.[43]

I first learned about high-dose vitamin D therapy for autoimmunity from my colleague, David Brownstein, MD, who had seen miraculous results with it. Cicero Coimbra, MD, PhD, has pioneered high-dose vitamin D for autoimmunity for over twenty years, laying a powerful foundation of scientific evidence, along with best practices for safe and effective use.

We start patients with autoimmunity at 10,000 IU of vitamin D daily in our practice. While vitamin D is essential for good health, it is also dangerous, as high doses can cause extreme elevations in calcium. We start patients at 10,000 IU and increase the dose from there depending upon their response and testing results. This must be done under medical supervision.

We pair vitamin D with K2 to ensure proper calcium metabolism. K2 directs calcium into bones and teeth, where it belongs, and away from arteries and soft tissues, where it causes problems.

We monitor vitamin D levels through testing and adjust dosing accordingly. Our target is at least 45 ng/mL.

For the high-dose vitamin D protocol we use in our practice, see the companion resources at stillmanmd.com/autoimmunity.

VITAMIN C

"The physician should give the patient vitamin C while they ponder the diagnosis."

—Frederick Klenner, MD

Dr. Klenner was right, which is why the high-dose vitamin C protocol is usually the first supplement protocol we share with our patients. Klenner used high-dose vitamin C and thiamine to treat patients with polio and multiple sclerosis in the mid-1900s with profound results. Whether you take high-dose vitamin C or a more modest dose, this is one of the supplements that patients most consistently see a benefit from.

Vitamin C creates the cross-links between collagen molecules that hold the body together.[44] Think of collagen as the bricks that constitute a building. Collagen without cross-links is like bricks without mortar. Without vitamin C, you fall apart.

The immune system needs vitamin C to eliminate pathogens and repair damaged tissues. The adrenal glands need it to produce stress hormones. The liver needs it to detoxify. Blood vessels need it to stay strong and flexible.

Modern food processing destroys vitamin C. Even fresh produce today has less vitamin C than it did a century ago due to soil depletion and early harvesting.[45] This is why we observe such dramatic improvements when we optimize vitamin C intake in our patients.

Our patients with autoimmunity (and many other issues) routinely report they notice a major improvement in their health and well-being with our vitamin C.

FRED'S STORY: VITAMIN C FOR REPAIR

Fred came to see us from Delaware. He had been struggling with chronic pain for years. His back pain was so severe that he was planning surgery. He had grandchildren he wanted to be able to pick up and play with.

Back surgeries usually fail. Patients start with one surgery and invariably come back for more over years or decades.

In our practice, we recommended vitamin C as a matter of course, not expecting it would impact his back pain specifically. To my surprise, he reported a few weeks later that it had reduced his pain from an 8 out of 10 to a 2 out of 10.

I was floored. This is why we recommend vitamin C to every patient in their first appointment. You never know what will respond until you try it.

It is critical to use a high-quality, properly buffered, fully-reacted vitamin C. Many products on the market are inferior and will not deliver the same results. As much as 30–70 percent of what is sold as vitamin C is not, in fact, vitamin C. I know this from testing products directly against each other. Our High-Dose Vitamin C Protocol, including the exact product we rely on, is in the companion resources at stillmanmd.com/autoimmunity.

DIGESTIVE ENZYMES

"All disease begins in the gut."

—Hippocrates

Nourishing our bodies starts with eating healthy, nourishing foods and taking essential supplements as needed. But what good are the nutrients in your food if your body cannot absorb them? Your body produces stomach acid, bile acid, and digestive enzymes to break down and absorb your food. Without these key ingredients, your food just sits in your stomach and rots. Without adequate stomach acid, patients often develop issues further down the digestive tract. Without adequate bile acids, they often wind up with low vitamin D levels and high bilirubin levels. Bilirubin is one of the key markers we covered in Chapter 5. Without adequate enzymes, you absorb less protein, which results in lower levels of essential amino acids that are needed to create and repair your cells, hormones, and neurotransmitters.

Digestive enzymes are critical to our well-being. As we age, our bodies produce fewer digestive enzymes.[46] Stress, processed food, and toxin exposure all impair enzyme production. Many of our patients with autoimmunity have severely compromised digestion. This is why we start here under medical supervision.

Lana, whom you met earlier (Chapter 5), was amazed by the effect of digestive enzymes. We started her on digestive enzymes before doing anything else. Within days, she reported that her bloating and abdominal pain had disappeared. She was shocked. She also noticed she was tolerating gluten and dairy better than she had in years.

In our practice, patients take one capsule with each meal under our supervision. We adjust based on meal size and individual response.

For exact products we use and complete protocols for complex digestive issues, see the Gut Healing Protocol in the companion resources at stillmanmd.com/autoimmunity.

DR. STILLMAN'S DETOX POWDER

I am a great believer in the healing power of plants and herbs. There are a handful of plants and herbs I have come to rely on in clinical practice. I tried to find a single product with the right ingredients, but could not find one. Instead of settling for a product I did not believe in, I created my own. Here are the ingredients:

- Kelp powder
- Alfalfa powder
- Chlorella powder
- Spirulina powder
- Dandelion root powder
- Milk thistle seed powder
- Beet root powder
- Ginger powder

Light therapy combined with the nutrients we have covered so far, plus Dr. Stillman's Detox Powder, forms the core of our approach. Daily use of these products can deliver remarkable results.

You can find out more about Dr. Stillman's Detox Powder in the companion resources at stillmanmd.com/autoimmunity.

Here is a story about how these simple daily tools can deliver exceptional results.

ANNETTE'S STORY: OVERCOMING FATIGUE, BRAIN FOG, AND POOR SLEEP

Annette came to us at age fifty-five with fatigue, brain fog, and poor sleep. She was struggling to lose weight. She had spent years as a patient of another functional medicine practice where she had taken overwhelming amounts of supplements. She was tired of taking so many pills each day and wanted to simplify. She had severe right knee pain that was keeping her from exercising. She wanted to keep up with her grandchildren and felt like her body was failing her.

We stopped all her prior supplements. We sent her a protocol built on these foundational supplements plus a few personalized additions based on her initial testing. We added light therapy for her knee pain.

A few months later, she reported that she was 90 percent better. She was sleeping well, she had an abundance of energy, and her memory and focus had markedly improved. Her knee pain disappeared within a week of starting daily light therapy.

She had spent years going to other doctors, taking massive doses of supplements, and feeling only marginally better for short periods of time.

We accomplished this with a much shorter list of supplements than she had been on, in only a few months. This is the power of micronutrients at the right dose, for the right duration, at the right frequency.

HOW TO ADJUST DOSES AND ROTATE PROTOCOLS

I never know who will respond to what, or what dose any given patient will need. I almost always recommend the supplements I have covered so far indefinitely.

Beyond these products and supplements, I add the following to round out a patient's plan of care. I often cycle these products in and out of someone's plan every six weeks. Why do I do this? Because six weeks is enough time to see if someone will clearly benefit from the vast majority of supplements. If a patient doesn't see a major benefit, we usually cut the supplement, unless we have a clear indication based on lab testing to continue it (see magnesium and fish oil, for example).

MAGNESIUM

"Magnesium deficiency can affect virtually every organ system of the body."

—Mildred Seelig, MD

Magnesium is required for hundreds of biochemical reactions in the body. It is essential for energy production, nerve function, muscle relaxation, and stress management.

Modern life depletes magnesium rapidly. The higher your stress levels, the faster you burn through magnesium. Modern farming and food processing methods lead to low levels of magnesium in our diets. The result is a modern epidemic of magnesium deficiency.

Low magnesium manifests as anxiety, insomnia, muscle cramps, constipation, heart and blood pressure issues, and more. When we restore magnesium levels in our patients, these symptoms often disappear.

This is why serum (blood) magnesium levels are part of our Repair Deficit Panel, covered in Chapter 5.

We give everyone magnesium for many reasons, but how much we give them varies widely. Depending on their diet, patients may already be eating anywhere from zero magnesium to over one gram of magnesium each day. Their absorption and losses vary widely as well. This is why we don't have a "one-size-fits-all" recommendation for magnesium.

We dose magnesium using a protocol available in the companion resources at stillmanmd.com/autoimmunity.

CHOLINE CITRATE

"Choline is essential for brain development, memory, and even mood regulation...yet an estimated 90 percent of Americans fall short on this key nutrient."

—David Perlmutter, MD[47]

I combine our powdered vitamin C with choline citrate and SOD B. I typically take magnesium at the same time, as choline assists with the absorption of magnesium and the correction of metabolic acidosis within cells.

Choline is a precursor to acetylcholine. Acetylcholine is the neurotransmitter of our parasympathetic nervous system, which is the part of our nervous system that allows us to relax, rest, and rejuvenate. Acetylcholine is also the main neurotransmitter of memory. Without choline, our memories deteriorate, and our nervous systems go into overdrive. With adequate choline, we can enter rest and digest mode to recover from exercise, injury, and illness, and achieve optimal brain function and cognition.

Our diets are extremely deficient in choline today due to modern food processing. This is why I take choline as a supplement. I also use it as a cognitive performance enhancer. I want all the brain power I can get.

RACHEL'S STORY: CHOLINE FOR MENTAL CLARITY

Rachel came to us struggling with what she described as a "tired but wired" feeling. She was exhausted but unable to relax. Many mothers in our practice know this combination well. You are running on empty, but your mind will not stop racing through everything you need to do for your family.

She noticed immediate effects from choline citrate on her mental clarity. When asked to rate her cognitive function on a scale of zero to ten, she said she had been at a one or two before. She described her cognitive function as "very bad" before choline citrate. With choline citrate, she rated herself at a six or seven. She was shocked by how much of a difference it made.

The effects don't last all day. Rachel finds they last one to two hours. But as she put it, "It's so much better than nothing." She takes it multiple times throughout the day when she needs clarity.

What struck me most was her comparison to prescription medications. She had previously used prescription drugs to improve her focus and mental clarity. She found choline citrate an equivalent, and at times better than the drugs. She noted that when the drugs stopped working, she could still rely on choline.

When I asked her to rate choline citrate as a supplement on a scale of zero to ten, she gave it a nine.

Individual results vary, of course. But Rachel's experience shows that choline citrate can provide meaningful cognitive support, especially for patients dealing with that "tired but wired" state.

Citrate helps to alkalinize the body. As we age, our bodies tend to become more acidic. We need to alkalinize to maintain optimal health and vitality. We measure acidity and alkalinity as pH. Your morning urinary pH is one of the predictors of early mortality, as we covered in Chapter 5. The lower it is, the more acidic you are, and the higher your risk of death. You can easily measure this with pH paper. The optimal urinary pH is approximately 7.0. Choline citrate helps us maintain a urinary pH of 7.0. Another benefit of our vitamin C is that it helps to correct pH, because it is correctly buffered. Most vitamin C available to consumers will drop their pH and can actually make them worse.

SOD B

I discovered the power of SOD B through my friend, Mary Rankin, who was so impressed with the product that she founded a company to bring it to practitioners and patients. We recorded a podcast together about her journey with autoimmunity. You can find it in the companion resources at stillmanmd.com/autoimmunity.

SOD B is a patented, clinically studied form of superoxide dismutase (SOD) derived from a proprietary melon variety. Superoxide dismutase is one of our primary antioxidant defenses. It neutralizes the oxidative stress that drives a repair deficit. Vitamin C works synergistically with SOD as part of the body's antioxidant network, helping to limit oxidative damage and support tissue repair.

Most oral SOD is destroyed by stomach acid before it can be absorbed. SOD B uses a protective coating that allows it to survive digestion and reach your cells intact. I combine SOD B with powdered vitamin C and liquid choline citrate for what I call "Dr. Stillman's Afternoon Pick-Me-Up."

FISH OIL

"Human beings evolved on a diet with a ratio of omega-6 to omega-3 essential fatty acids of approximately 1:1, whereas today this ratio is 15:1 to 17:1."[48]

—Artemis Simopoulos, MD

Fish oil has been well-documented to improve brain health and cognitive function. It has been shown to reduce your risk of dementia.[49] It has been shown to improve brain health in children. The omega-3 fatty acids in fish oil are essential building blocks for cell membranes throughout the body, particularly in the brain and nervous system.

Fish oil also has powerful anti-inflammatory effects. This is particularly important for people with autoimmunity, where chronic inflammation is a central feature of repair deficit and therefore the disease itself.

The quality of fish oil matters tremendously. Many products are rancid, contaminated with mercury or other toxins, or processed into what one of my friends calls "Frankenstein fish oil." We use only the highest quality fish oil that has been tested for purity and potency.

Not everyone needs a fish oil supplement. Some should, in fact, avoid them. For our complete guide on fish oil, see the Fish, Fish Oil, and Autoimmunity guide in the companion resources at stillmanmd.com/autoimmunity.

ADVANCED AND HIGH-DOSE PROTOCOLS

Beyond these products and supplements, we have a growing number of advanced protocols we share with our patients. These require more attention to detail, more time, and they can come with unpleasant side effects as the body heals. This is why we do not start with them. They are not for everyone. We recommend medical supervision in implementing these protocols, although their ingredients are all available over the counter and have been used safely for generations.

In our practice, we typically introduce advanced protocols in six-week rotations. We add one protocol at a time, monitor the response, and then decide whether to continue, adjust, or move on to the next intervention.

The three nutrients we start patients on high doses of are vitamin C, methylsulfonylmethane (MSM), and iodine. We typically use them in that order.

The full protocols for each of these are available online at stillmanmd.com/autoimmunity. If you want exact details, you can access them there.

I recommend starting with the Vitamin C Protocol first, but since we already discussed vitamin C in the Foundational Five, we will move on to MSM.

THE MSM PROTOCOL

"MSM is a naturally occurring sulfur compound found in our bodies and in many foods. It is as safe as water."

—Stanley Jacob, MD

MSM stands for methylsulfonylmethane. We typically start patients on low doses throughout the day and work up to twenty grams daily over several days. You have to work up to this dose slowly, as some patients will have side effects with less than a gram. We use the protocol to determine who can tolerate it well and who is sensitive.

Many patients see dramatic improvements in pain, inflammation, and overall well-being with MSM. The key is working up to an adequate dose. Most people who try MSM never get close to therapeutic dosing and miss out on the benefits.

This is one reason why most people have never heard of MSM.

MSM is one of our most powerful therapeutics. For the complete MSM protocol, see the companion resources at stillmanmd.com/autoimmunity.

THE HIGH-DOSE IODINE PROTOCOL

"When I was a medical student, iodine in the form of potassium iodide was the universal medicine. Nobody knew what it did, but it did something and did something good."

—Albert Szent-Györgyi, Nobel laureate

Iodine is essential for thyroid function, but it does so much more. Iodine plays a role in all of your body's cells for optimal health. It supports breast health, prostate health, brain health, and overall hormonal balance. It helps the body eliminate toxic halogens like fluoride, chlorine, and bromine.

Most people today are severely deficient in iodine. Our environment is full of toxic halides that displace iodine from our bodies. Processed food is devoid of iodine. The result is that patients are often amazed by the results they see with even low doses of iodine.

High-dose iodine requires medical supervision and monitoring. Some people experience detox symptoms as they clear toxic halogens. Patients can and do develop hyperthyroidism on high-dose iodine. We have a discussion with each patient regarding the risks and benefits of high-dose iodine before starting it. We may defer using it or patients may decide against it. This is not a protocol to attempt without guidance.

For the complete High-Dose Iodine Protocol, see the companion resources at stillmanmd.com/autoimmunity.

COMPANION RESOURCES FOR SUPPLEMENT PROTOCOLS

The companion resources at stillmanmd.com/autoimmunity include "Supplements I Take Every Day," our High-Dose Vitamin C, Vitamin D, MSM, and Iodine Protocols, the Gut Healing Protocol, and more information on Dr. Stillman's Detox Powder.

BIOIDENTICAL HORMONES

"Hormones are the messengers that tell our cells what to do. Without adequate hormones, we cannot maintain health."

—Thierry Hertoghe, MD

Bioidentical hormones are a key component of our framework for treating autoimmunity. Why am I such a believer in hormones?

First, I have seen the evidence in my practice. Bioidentical hormones are life-giving, life-saving medications. In case after case, bioidentical hormones delivered results that nothing else could. Patients were saved from misery by a few drops of oil, a dab of cream, or a tiny injection.

Second, we live in a hormone-disrupted world. From microplastics to pesticides to heavy metals, we are exposed to more and more hormone-disrupting compounds in our environment. Optimizing our hormones is vital to optimal health in this toxic world.

Third, hormone levels decline as we age, and there are significant benefits to maintaining youthful levels. The media have trumped up the risks, despite the fact that many studies have shown benefits that outweigh risks.

What are bioidentical hormones? They are hormones that are exactly identical to what the body makes naturally. We use them in our practice every day. When most people say "hormones," they usually do not mean bioidentical hormones. They are typically referring to synthetic hormones that are certainly dangerous.

Most doctors are ignorant of the true literature on this topic. They do not understand the distinction between bioidentical hormones and synthetic hormones. They are wrong. Bioidentical hormones are incredibly beneficial for patients. The literature continues to show that they reduce our risk of major illness and death, while improving our quality of life.[50]

Are bioidentical hormones right for everyone? Professionally, I believe that everyone, at some point in their life and for some period of time, will benefit from them. Exactly what, when, and for how long is up to you to determine with your practitioner.

We prescribe progesterone, estrogen, testosterone, DHEA, and thyroid hormone. These are the key hormones we see transforming lives time and again in our practice.

Here is a story about hormones and autoimmunity from our practice.

BETH'S STORY: LICHEN SCLEROSUS AND BIOIDENTICAL HORMONES

Beth came to us with an autoimmune skin condition called lichen sclerosus a few years ago. Lichen sclerosus affects the skin around the vagina and anus, and can extend up to the abdomen. The skin scars down, narrowing the vaginal opening. Sex becomes painful or even impossible. She noted her symptoms started shortly after receiving a series of vaccines.

We tried everything. We personalized her supplements, started light therapy patches, and even used UV light. Steroid creams from her dermatologist and gynecologist did not work.

Finally, we started bioidentical hormone oils on the affected skin, and within a few months, her symptoms went into remission. Her condition flared a few times over the next few years, and she added a topical gel that resolved her flares.

Beyond her skin, Beth has more energy, is losing weight, and is in better spirits than she has been in years. She feels great. She loves her bioidentical hormones.

Bioidentical hormones help the body resist disease and

repair the damage of daily life. There is an abundance of evidence that bioidentical hormones can help us overcome autoimmunity. This is why we use bioidentical hormones in our practice.

Bioidentical hormones require medical supervision and prescription. They are not something you can implement on your own. They are incredibly powerful tools that can make the difference between struggling and thriving.

For complete guides on bioidentical hormones, see the companion resources at stillmanmd.com/autoimmunity. You'll find everything Beth used to get her lichen sclerosus into remission in the companion resources, including guides on treatments for autoimmune skin disorders, bioidentical hormones in autoimmunity, menopause, and hormone balancing before, during, and after menopause.

REPURPOSED DRUGS

"One sometimes finds what one is not looking for."

—Sir Alexander Fleming[51]

Most drugs have many effects, but are only prescribed for one of them. Erectile dysfunction drugs were originally studied to treat high blood pressure. The male study participants noticed an unexpected side effect, and researchers repurposed the drugs quickly. Now, hardly anyone takes these drugs for high blood pressure.

We are increasingly using repurposed drugs to treat autoimmune diseases. Anti-parasitics, anti-malarials, and other medications originally developed for completely different purposes can have profound effects on autoimmunity.

PETER'S STORY: RECOVERY WITH IVERMECTIN AND METHYLENE BLUE

Peter came to see us in July 2024. He was struggling with chest pain, anxiety, and panic attacks. He had lost the stamina to even ride his bicycle. He had been to many other physicians before he came to see us.

His first hair tissue test showed one of the highest levels of nickel we have ever seen in the practice. We started personalized supplementation with an extremely high dose of zinc and he saw significant improvements over the next few months.

After six months of supplementation, he started ivermectin and methylene blue and was amazed by the improvements he saw. Ivermectin is an anti-parasitic. Methylene blue is generally only used rarely in intensive care settings for shock. Both have been repurposed as outpatient medications for the treatment of a wide range of conditions.

Between personalized supplementation and repurposed drugs, Peter achieved a complete resolution of his symptoms.

Most of the drugs being repurposed for autoimmunity have some kind of effect on the immune system. Anti-parasitics have complex effects on immune balance in addition to eliminating parasites. Both properties would potentially explain the results patients often report when using these drugs to treat autoimmunity.

We do not always start with drugs, because they do not usually help us fix a repair deficit. They can augment or modulate the immune response in such a way as to help resolve the inflammation associated with autoimmunity. We use them on a case-by-case basis.

One thing is clear about repurposed drugs. They can work wonders in autoimmunity. The key is finding the right agent, using it at the right dose, and for the right duration of time.

Repurposed drugs require medical supervision and a prescription. For our complete guide on repurposed drugs for autoimmunity, see the free resources at stillmanmd.com/autoimmunity.

COMPANION RESOURCES FOR HORMONES AND ADVANCED THERAPEUTICS

I have prepared companion resources on hormones, repurposed drugs, and more advanced therapeutics at stillmanmd.com/autoimmunity.

THE GOOD, BETTER, BEST HIERARCHY

I usually share this material with patients over a period of months. This largely depends upon patients and how much they can handle. They may not have enough time, energy, or mental bandwidth to do more than a few of the things I have outlined here. They may tackle the whole "stack" of supplements in under a week. Don't feel like you have to do everything at once. Often the patients who take a steadier, more consistent approach, adopting a few habits or supplements every week rather than all at once, get the best results. Slow and steady may be better than all at once.

Good means getting started with the supplements and products in the order I have presented them, with proper medical clearance (of course). Don't assume you need all of these supplements to thrive. Most of our patients settle on five to ten that they fall in love with after experiencing them.

Better means adding one supplement or product listed here at a time, until you have tried each for at least six weeks. Six weeks of daily use is almost always enough time to determine how much a given supplement or product will move the needle in your case. There are exceptions to this. This is where education and guidance become valuable.

Best means high-dose supplement protocols (vitamin C, MSM, and iodine, for example), personalized supplement protocols based on testing, bioidentical hormones, and repurposed drugs when indicated. This requires working directly with a qualified practitioner.

Remember that some of the most compelling case studies in this book had nothing to do with Therapeutics. Ashlee recovered her health in Hawaii with diet and lifestyle changes alone. Jim restored his gut with dietary changes and a few carefully chosen supplements. Teresa just ditched her sunscreen and sunglasses. Kelly was shocked by how much better her headaches were when she reduced her electrosmog exposure. Therapeutics build on the foundation set by daily implementation of Essentials and avoidance of Hazards.

YOUR NEXT STEP

Your next step depends on where you are.

If you are ready to try some of the supplements and products mentioned here, download the companion resources "Healing with Light" and "Supplements I Take Every Day" from stillmanmd.com/autoimmunity. As always, seek appropriate medical supervision.

If you have questions about Therapeutics, submit a question at stillmanmd.com/autoimmunity. I'll do my best to answer them in one of our Q&A's.

COMPANION RESOURCES FOR CHAPTER 6

The Chapter 6 companion resources at stillmanmd.com/autoimmunity bring together everything you need to implement the therapeutics discussed in this chapter. You will find:

- "Healing with Light" and the podcasts about light therapy with Kathleen Horstmeyer and Meredith Oke.
- "Supplements I Take Every Day" and "Dr. Stillman's Detox Powder."
- High-dose supplement protocols for Vitamin C, Vitamin D, MSM, and iodine.
- "Gut Repair Essentials: Our 5-Step Process."
- Guide to bioidentical hormones, including exact products and protocols we use in our practice for thyroid, estrogen, progesterone, and more.
- Advanced therapeutics, such as repurposed drugs, ozone, hyperbaric oxygen, and more.

CHAPTER 7

The End of Autoimmunity

"For I know the plans I have for you, declares the Lord, plans for welfare and not for evil, to give you a future and a hope."

—JEREMIAH 29:11

If you have made it this far, then you know that practically everything about modern life, from the fluoride in toothpaste to the chemicals in non-stick cookware to the aluminum in deodorant to the pesticides in food, is playing a role in our epidemic of autoimmunity.

How can we possibly stop, let alone reverse, this epidemic? What does a future without autoimmunity look like?

It looks a lot like the past.

We need to keep our skies clear and our indoor air pristine. We need to keep our homes and offices healthy, which means free of mold, toxic chemicals, and allergens like dust mites. This means better construction and circulation through our HVAC systems.

We need to restore the integrity of our water. We must protect our rivers, streams, lakes, and oceans from pollution. We must protect our aquifers, wells, and ground water.

We need to return to local, organic agriculture. You should know the person who planted, picked, and transported your food to wherever you bought it. The food should be kept in glass or wax paper, never plastic or aluminum. It should be cooked within a few days of purchase. It should be eaten with friends or family, rather than alone.

We need to somehow reduce the burden of heavy metals and toxic chemicals in our environment. While reducing sources of pollution will help, it will do nothing to remove the heavy metals and "forever chemicals" that are already in the biosphere. To reduce the global burden of these toxins, we will need to eliminate or sequester them. I have no idea how, exactly, but governments, corporations, and individuals must find ways to destroy, sequester, or remove toxins from the biosphere.

We need to eliminate electrosmog as much as possible. This means going back to landlines and wired headphones, computer keyboards, and more. The world will be connected by fiber-optic cable.

Wireless communication in particular is fraying the social fabric of our society. People are more connected, and yet more lonely, than ever. The internet is a wonderful thing, but being constantly connected wirelessly is disconnecting us from one another in reality. This is eroding the mental health of our most vulnerable—the young and the elderly. We need to return to a culture of in-person socialization.

The future I hope for is one with minimal technology and electrical consumption, with hyper-efficient computers that we use during the day, and then shut down each night. It is a future of wholesome, healthy, fresh food that is locally grown and consumed. It is a future of protected water resources that are of the highest quality. It is a future where mothers and babies can eat tuna without worrying about losing their minds due to mercury exposure. It is a future where everyone is connected by fiber-optic cable, rather than wireless devices. It is a future where we have gone back to what was good about the past, and kept what we love about the present.

How can we create this future? These are complex questions and I certainly don't have all the answers.

What I do know is that it starts with each of us taking ownership of and responsibility for not only our health, but for how we treat one another and live our daily lives.

I believe it starts with what I included in this book.

You hold in your hands secrets that took me twenty years to learn and more than I care to admit in training, travel, and mentorship to obtain.

My question to you is, "What will you do with it?"

WHAT'S ACTUALLY POSSIBLE?

Let me be direct about what you can expect, because I believe strongly that we should always state the facts and tell the truth.

Between January and December 2025, we surveyed every patient who completed a program or membership at our practice. Only a handful did not respond. The 103 who did respond reported an average overall improvement of 67 percent in general well-being. By specific domain, they reported their mood improved 75 percent, stamina improved 71 percent, cognition improved 71 percent, digestion improved 70 percent, energy improved 70 percent, and sleep improved 70 percent. Our patient satisfaction is in the top 10 percent of medical practices.[52]

These were self-reported and subjective improvements. We do not offer miracle cures, and we don't have a "silver bullet" for autoimmunity.

What we do have is a clearly defined process and framework that our patients find great value in. These are life-changing improvements. Patients went from barely functioning to living full, productive lives.

Don't take my word for it. Hear it in their own words. In the companion resources online, I include links to podcasts I have recorded with patients like Meredith and Emily, and friends and colleagues like Amy, Ashlee, and Jim. I encourage you to listen to these stories for inspiration and education.

YOUR NEXT STEP

You've seen what's possible. Now you need a plan that fits your story, your values, and your season of life.

If you'd like our help determining the best program of care for you, then your next step is simple:

1. Open your browser.
2. Go to stillmanmd.com/autoimmunity.
3. Book an assessment with our team.

During this assessment, we will:

- Listen to your story, symptoms, and goals.
- Review what you've already tried.
- Recommend the level of support that fits your values, time, and resources.
- Outline clear next steps so you leave knowing exactly what to do next.

You are not committing to a program or becoming a patient by booking this call. You are committing to clarity. If you're worried about your fit for our programs, cost, or location, know that we work with and refer to practitioners all over the world. We'll do our best to help you find the best care for you, even if that's not at our practice.

Our team sets aside a limited number of these assessments each week, so book yours today.

Go to stillmanmd.com/autoimmunity and book your assessment. Here's a QR code if that's easier:

IF YOU ARE A PRACTITIONER

If you're a practitioner or coach, we would like to collaborate with you to make this future a reality. We're building a network of practitioners and coaches who share our values and our approach to medicine. You can train in our method and learn about our referral process. If you'd like to partner with us, go to the "For Practitioners" section at stillmanmd.com/autoimmunity. There you can:

- Download the more technical versions of the Repair Deficit Panel and HTMA guides
- Learn about practitioner training opportunities
- Ask to be notified when our practitioner directory and training cohorts open

- Learn how to join our practitioner network so we can refer patients or clients to you

A FINAL WORD

I hope that you'll stay connected to me beyond this book. Go to stillmanmd.com/autoimmunity and subscribe to our newsletter. That's where I'll keep you up to date on all things autoimmunity, including opportunities to get involved in creating the kind of future we all hope for, where the epidemic of autoimmunity is history, a cautionary tale about hubris, and a story of redeeming our birthright of good health.

Until next time, be well,
Dr. Stillman

P.S. If this book was useful to you, would you be so kind as to leave a review wherever you purchased, listened to, or read it? Your review may help someone else who is sick and searching find their way to this information.

Acknowledgments

First, to my wife, Michelle. Your love humbles and inspires me.

Second, to my parents. To my mother, for giving me a deep and abiding love for humanity. To my father, for teaching me to outwork everyone else and to live based on my principles.

Third, to Mimi and Pops. This book wouldn't have been possible without your support.

Fourth, to my mentors, past and present, who passed on their art to me. Each of you gave me priceless secrets from a lifetime of practice, and for this, I am eternally grateful. I have truly stood on the shoulders of giants.

Fifth, to Amy, Tori, Kenna, and Christy, I don't know what I would do without you. You make the practice what it is.

Sixth, to Kathleen, Richard, Thora, Ashlee, and my whole team at LifeWave. You make this a lot less lonely and a lot more fun.

Seventh, to my patients, customers, and to anyone who helped me pay my bills. I can't thank you enough.

Last, but not least, to Alex and Leila Hormozi and the team at Acquisition.com, I would not have had the time and resources to write this book without your guidance and input.

Notes

1 Witebsky E, Rose NR, Ter Borg M, Hargrove M. Origins and history of autoimmunity—a brief review. *Immunol Rev.* 2022;308(1):9-24. doi:10.1111/imr.13098.

2 Rose NR, Mackay IR, eds. *The Autoimmune Diseases.* 5th ed. Elsevier; 2014.

3 Lerner A, Jeremias P, Matthias T. The world incidence and prevalence of autoimmune diseases is increasing. *Int J Celiac Dis.* 2015;3(4):151-155. doi:10.12691/ijcd-3-4-8.

4 Cooper GS, Stroehla BC. The epidemiology of autoimmune diseases. *Autoimmun Rev.* 2003;2(3):119-125. doi:10.1016/S1568-9972(03)00006-5.

5 Platts-Mills TAE. The allergy epidemics: 1870–2010. *J Allergy Clin Immunol.* 2015;136(1):3-13. doi:10.1016/j.jaci.2015.03.048; Cowan T. *Vaccines, Autoimmunity, and the Changing Nature of Childhood Illness.* Chelsea Green Publishing; 2018.

6 Dinse GE, Parks CG, Weinberg CR, Co CA, Wilkerson J, Zeldin DC, et al. Increasing prevalence of antinuclear antibodies in the United States. *Arthritis Rheumatol.* 2020;72(6):1026-1035. doi:10.1002/art.41214; Berhan Y, Waernbaum I, Lind T, Möllsten A, Dahlquist G. Thirty years of prospective nationwide incidence of childhood type 1 diabetes: the accelerating increase by time tends to level off in Sweden. *Diabetes.* 2011;60(2):577-581. doi:10.2337/db10-0813; NIH Office of Autoimmune Disease Research. *NIH-Wide Strategic Plan for Autoimmune Disease Research.* National Institutes of Health; 2025. Accessed May 7, 2026. https://orwh.od.nih.gov/sites/orwh/files/docs/ORWH_OADR_StrategicPlan_2025_508.pdf; National Health Council. A major health crisis: the alarming rise of autoimmune disease. Published March 28, 2024. Accessed May 7, 2026. https://www.nationalhealthcouncil.org/blog/a-major-health-crisis-the-alarming-rise-of-autoimmune-disease/; Lerner A, Jeremias P, Matthias T. The world incidence and prevalence of autoimmune diseases is increasing. *Int J Celiac Dis.* 2015;3(4):151-155. doi:10.12691/ijcd-3-4-8.

7 Mold M, Chmielecka A, Ramirez Rodriguez MR, Thom F, Linhart C, King A, et al. Aluminium in brain tissue in multiple sclerosis. *Int J Environ Res Public Health.* 2018;15(8):1777. doi:10.3390/ijerph15081777; Exley C. *Imagine You Are an Aluminum Atom: Discussions with Mr. Aluminum.* Skyhorse Publishing; 2020.

8 Stahl T, Falk S, Rohrbeck A, Georgii S. Migration of aluminum from food contact materials to food—a health risk for consumers? Part I of III: exposure to aluminum, release of aluminum, tolerable weekly intake (TWI), toxicological effects of aluminum, study design, and methods. *Environ Sci Eur.* 2017;29(1). doi:10.1186/s12302-017-0116-y; Exley C. *Imagine You Are an Aluminum Atom: Discussions with Mr. Aluminum.* Skyhorse Publishing; 2020.

9 Kharrazian D. Exposure to environmental toxins and autoimmune conditions. *Integr Med (Encinitas).* 2021;20(2):20-24.

10 Abu-Shakra M, Buskila D, Shoenfeld Y. Molecular mimicry between host and pathogen: examples from parasites and implication. *Immunol Lett.* 1999;67(2):147-152. doi:10.1016/s0165-2478(99)00004-8.

11 Byliński Ł, Kostelecka K, Woliński F, Duda P, Góra J, Granat M, et al. Aluminium in the human brain: routes of penetration, toxicity, and resulting complications. *Int J Mol Sci.* 2023;24(8):7228. doi:10.3390/ijms24087228; Miller CS. Toxicant-induced loss of tolerance—an emerging theory of disease? *Environ Health Perspect.* 1997;105(suppl 2):445-453. doi:10.1289/ehp.97105s2445.

12 Medzhitov R. Origin and physiological roles of inflammation. *Nature.* 2008;454:428-435. doi:10.1038/nature07201; Furman D, Campisi J, Verdin E, Carrera-Bastos P, Targ S, Franceschi C, et al. Chronic inflammation in the etiology of disease across the life span. *Nat Med.* 2019;25:1822-1832. doi:10.1038/s41591-019-0675-0.

13 Davidson A, Diamond B. Autoimmune diseases. *N Engl J Med.* 2001;345(5):340-350. doi:10.1056/NEJM200108023450506.

14 I have expressed toxic metal levels in terms of mcg% in the text, while the images show these levels in mg%. This is so that in the audiobook, I do not have to say "zero point" over and over again. The amount is the same; all that has changed is the position of the decimal point.

15 Takayama A, Takeshima T, Yamazaki H, Kamitani T, Shimizu S, Fukuhara S, et al. Resting respiration rate predicts all-cause mortality in older outpatients. *Aging Clin Exp Res.* 2022;34:1697-1705. doi:10.1007/s40520-022-02104-0; Baumert M, Linz D, Stone K, McEvoy RD, Cummings S, Redline S, et al. Mean nocturnal respiratory rate predicts cardiovascular and all-cause mortality in community-dwelling older men and women. *Eur Respir J.* 2019;54(1):1802175. doi:10.1183/13993003.02175-2018.

16 Bogdan C. Nitric oxide and the immune response. *Nat Immunol.* 2001;2:907-916. doi:10.1038/ni1001-907.

17 Drager LF, Togeiro SM, Polotsky VY, Lorenzi-Filho G. Obstructive sleep apnea: a cardiometabolic risk in obesity and the metabolic syndrome. *J Am Coll Cardiol.* 2013;62(7):569-576. doi:10.1016/j.jacc.2013.05.045; Hassan AK. Relation between mouth breather patients and their sexual activities, pilot study. *J Oral Health Dent Sci.* 2019;3(2):201.

18 Disanto G, Morahan JM, Barnett MH, Giovannoni G, Ramagopalan SV. Multiple sclerosis: risk factors and their interactions. *CNS Neurol Disord Drug Targets.* 2012;11(5):545-555. doi:10.2174/187152712801661266.

19 Hedström AK, Åkerstedt T, Hillert J, Olsson T, Alfredsson L. Shift work at young age is associated with increased risk for multiple sclerosis. *Ann Neurol.* 2011;70(5):733-741. doi:10.1002/ana.22597.

20 Tähkämö L, Partonen T, Pesonen AK. Systematic review of light exposure impact on human circadian rhythm. *Chronobiol Int.* 2019;36(2):151-170. doi:10.1080/07420528.2018.1527773.

21 Klepeis NE, Nelson WC, Ott WR, Robinson JP, Tsang AM, Switzer P, et al. The National Human Activity Pattern Survey (NHAPS): a resource for assessing exposure to environmental pollutants. *J Expo Sci Environ Epidemiol.* 2001;11:231-252. doi:10.1038/sj.jea.7500165.

22 Hönigsmann H. History of phototherapy in dermatology. *Photochem Photobiol Sci.* 2013;12:16-21. doi:10.1039/C2PP25120E.

23 Srour B, Fezeu LK, Kesse-Guyot E, Allès B, Méjean C, Andrianasolo RM, et al. Ultra-processed food intake and risk of cardiovascular disease: prospective cohort study (NutriNet-Santé). *BMJ.* 2019;365:l1451. doi:10.1136/bmj.l1451; Narula N, Wong ECL, Dehghan M, Mente A, Rangarajan S, Lanas F, et al. Association of ultra-processed food intake with risk of inflammatory bowel disease: prospective cohort study. *BMJ.* 2021;374:n1554. doi:10.1136/bmj.n1554; Rico-Campà A, Martínez-González MA, Alvarez-Alvarez I, de Deus Mendonça R, de la Fuente-Arrillaga C, Gómez-Donoso C, et al. Association between consumption of ultra-processed foods and all cause mortality: SUN prospective cohort study. *BMJ.* 2019;365:l1949. doi:10.1136/bmj.l1949.

24 Zuo Y, Lu X, Wang X, Sooranna SR, Tao L, Chen S, et al. High-dose aluminum exposure further alerts immune phenotype in aplastic anemia patients. *Biol Trace Elem Res.* 2021;199(5):1743-1753. doi:10.1007/s12011-020-02313-6; Mold M, Chmielecka A, Ramirez Rodriguez MR, Thom F, Linhart C, King A, et al. Aluminium in brain tissue in multiple sclerosis. *Int J Environ Res Public Health.* 2018;15(8):1777. doi:10.3390/ijerph15081777.

25 Exley C. Human exposure to aluminium. *Environ Sci Process Impacts.* 2013;15(10):1807-1816. doi:10.1039/C3EM00374D.

26 Lindqvist PG, Epstein E, Nielsen K, Landin-Olsson M, Ingvar C, Olsson H. Avoidance of sun exposure as a risk factor for major causes of death: a competing risk analysis of the melanoma in southern Sweden cohort. *J Intern Med.* 2016;280(4):375-387. doi:10.1111/joim.12496.

27 Rosso S, Sera F, Segnan N, Zanetti R. Sun exposure prior to diagnosis is associated with improved survival in melanoma patients: results from a long-term follow-up study of Italian patients. *Eur J Cancer.* 2008;44(9):1275-1281. doi:10.1016/j.ejca.2008.03.009.

28 Huncharek M, Kupelnick B. Use of topical sunscreens and the risk of malignant melanoma: a meta-analysis of 9067 patients from 11 case-control studies. *Am J Public Health.* 2002;92(7):1173-1177. doi:10.2105/AJPH.92.7.1173.

29 Berwick M, Armstrong BK, Ben-Porat L, Fine J, Kricker A, Eberle C, et al. Sun exposure and mortality from melanoma. *J Natl Cancer Inst.* 2005;97(3):195-202. doi:10.1093/jnci/dji019.

30 Guth S, Hüser S, Roth A, Degen G, Diel P, Edlund K, et al. Toxicity of fluoride: critical evaluation of evidence for human developmental neurotoxicity in epidemiological studies, animal experiments and in vitro analyses. *Arch Toxicol.* 2020;94(5):1375-1415. doi:10.1007/s00204-020-02725-2; Choi AL, Sun G, Zhang Y, Grandjean P. Developmental fluoride neurotoxicity: a systematic review and meta-analysis. *Environ Health Perspect.* 2012;120(10):1362-1368. doi:10.1289/ehp.1104912; Bashash M, Thomas D, Hu H, Martinez-Mier EA, Sanchez BN, Basu N, et al. Prenatal fluoride exposure and cognitive outcomes in children at 4 and 6–12 years of age in Mexico. *Environ Health Perspect.* 2017;125(9):097017. doi:10.1289/EHP655; Perera T, Ranasinghe S, Alles N, Waduge R. Effect of fluoride on major organs with the different time of exposure in rats. *Environ Health Prev Med.* 2018;23(1):17. doi:10.1186/s12199-018-0707-2; Johnston NR, Strobel SA. Principles of fluoride toxicity and the cellular response: a review. *Arch Toxicol.* 2020;94(4):1051-1069. doi:10.1007/s00204-020-02687-5.

31 Rubin RL. Drug-induced lupus. *Expert Opin Drug Saf.* 2015;14(3):361-378. doi:10.1517/14740338.2015.995089; Conrad K, Röber N, Andrade LEC, Mahler M. The clinical relevance of anti-DFS70 autoantibodies. *Clin Rev Allergy Immunol.* 2017;52(2):202-216. doi:10.1007/s12016-016-8564-5; Gherardi RK, Eidi H, Crépeaux G, Authier FJ, Cadusseau J. Biopersistence and brain translocation of aluminum adjuvants of vaccines. *Front Neurol.* 2015;6:4. doi:10.3389/fneur.2015.00004; Tomljenovic L, Shaw CA. Mechanisms of aluminum adjuvant toxicity and autoimmunity in pediatric populations. *Lupus.* 2012;21(2). doi:10.1177/0961203311430221; Shoenfeld Y, Agmon-Levin N. "ASIA"—autoimmune/inflammatory syndrome induced by adjuvants. *J Autoimmun.* 2011;36(1):4-8. doi:10.1016/j.jaut.2010.07.003; Segal Y, Shoenfeld Y. Vaccine-induced autoimmunity: the role of molecular mimicry and immune crossreaction. *Cell Mol Immunol.* 2018;15:586-594. doi:10.1038/cmi.2017.151.

32 Miller CS. Toxicant-induced loss of tolerance. *Addiction.* 2001;96(1):115-137. doi:10.1046/j.1360-0443.2001.9611159.x.

33 Song H, Fang F, Tomasson G, Arnberg FK, Mataix-Cols D, Fernández de la Cruz L, et al. Association of stress-related disorders with subsequent autoimmune disease. *JAMA.* 2018;319(23):2388-2400. doi:10.1001/jama.2018.7028.

34 Porter CK, Cash BD, Pimentel M, Akinseye A, Riddle MS. Risk of inflammatory bowel disease following a diagnosis of irritable bowel syndrome. *BMC Gastroenterol.* 2012;12:55. doi:10.1186/1471-230X-12-55; Song H, Zhou Y, Liu S, Zhang Q, Zhang S, Zhu S, et al. Long-term risk of inflammatory bowel disease in patients with irritable bowel syndrome: the cross-sectional and longitudinal relationship. *J Gastroenterol.* 2026;61:139-149. doi:10.1007/s00535-025-02304-1.

35 Marrie RA, Cohen J, Stuve O, Trojano M, Sørensen PS, Reingold S, et al. A systematic review of the incidence and prevalence of comorbidity in multiple sclerosis. *Mult Scler.* 2015;21(3). doi:10.1177/1352458514564491; Levinthal DJ, Rahman A, Nusrat S, O'Leary M, Heyman R, Bielefeldt K. Adding to the burden: gastrointestinal symptoms and syndromes in multiple sclerosis. *Mult Scler Int.* 2013:319201. doi:10.1155/2013/319201.

36 Wolfe F, Petri M, Alarcón GS, Goldman J, Chakravarty EF, Katz RS, et al. Fibromyalgia, systemic lupus erythematosus (SLE), and evaluation of SLE activity. *J Rheumatol.* 2009;36(1):82-88. doi:10.3899/jrheum.080212; Wang Q, Chaudhary P, Chang Y, Garg M. Fibromyalgia as a potential initial presentation for autoimmune conditions. Abstract presented at: ACR Convergence 2024; November 14–19, 2024; Washington, DC. https://acrabstracts.org/abstract/fibromyalgia-as-a-potential-initial-presentation-for-autoimmune-conditions/; Weir PT, Harlan GA, Nkoy FL, Jones SS, Hegmann KT, Gren LH, et al. The incidence of fibromyalgia and its associated comorbidities: a population-based retrospective cohort study based on international classification of diseases, 9th revision codes. *J Clin Rheumatol.* 2006;12(3):124-128. doi:10.1097/01.rhu.0000221817.46231.18.

37 Park N-H, Kang Y-E, Yoon J-H, Ahn Y-C, Lee E-J, Park B-J, et al. Comparative study for fatigue prevalence in subjects with diseases: a systematic review and meta-analysis. *Sci Rep.* 2024;14:23348. doi:10.1038/s41598-024-74683-z; Wirth KJ, Löhn M. Myalgic encephalomyelitis/chronic fatigue syndrome (ME/CFS) and comorbidities: linked by vascular pathomechanisms and vasoactive mediators? *Medicina.* 2023;59(5):978. doi:10.3390/medicina59050978; Batham J, Dwyer J, Eaton-Fitch N, Marshall-Gradisnik S. Autoimmunity's enigmatic role: exploring the connection with myalgic encephalomyelitis/chronic fatigue syndrome. *BMC Immunol.* 2024;25:62. doi:10.1186/s12865-024-00657-5.

38 Shani U, David P, Strosberg IB, Regev O, Yihia M, Ben-Shabat N, et al. Mortality in antinuclear antibody-positive patients with and without rheumatologic immune-related disorders: a large-scale population-based study. *Medicina.* 2025;61(1):60. doi:10.3390/medicina61010060.

39 Malavolta M, Piacenza F, Basso A, Giacconi R, Costarelli L, Mocchegiani E. Serum copper to zinc ratio: relationship with aging and health status. *Mech Ageing Dev.* 2015;151:93-100. doi:10.1016/j.mad.2015.01.004.

40 Lawton RI, Sabatini BL, Hochbaum DR. Longevity, demographic characteristics, and socio-economic status are linked to triiodothyronine levels in the general population. *Proc Natl Acad Sci U S A.* 2024;121(2):e2308652121. doi:10.1073/pnas.2308652121.

41 Davis DR, Epp MD, Riordan HD. Changes in USDA food composition data for 43 garden crops, 1950 to 1999. *J Am Coll Nutr.* 2004;23(6):669-682. doi:10.1080/07315724.2004.10719409; Bhardwaj RL, Parashar A, Parewa HP, Vyas L. An alarming decline in the nutritional quality of foods: the biggest challenge for future generations' health. *Foods.* 2024;13(6):877. doi:10.3390/foods13060877.

42 Hamblin MR. Mechanisms and applications of the anti-inflammatory effects of photobiomodulation. *AIMS Biophys.* 2017;4(3):337-361. doi:10.3934/biophy.2017.3.337.

43 Aranow C. Vitamin D and the immune system. *J Investig Med.* 2011;59(6):881-886. doi:10.2310/JIM.0b013e31821b8755.

44 Murad S, Grove D, Lindberg KA, Reynolds G, Sivarajah A, Pinnell SR. Regulation of collagen synthesis by ascorbic acid. *Proc Natl Acad Sci U S A.* 1981;78(5):2879-2882. doi:10.1073/pnas.78.5.2879.

45 Davis DR. Declining fruit and vegetable nutrient composition: what is the evidence? *HortScience.* 2009;44(1):15-19. doi:10.21273/HORTSCI.44.1.15.

46 Drozdowski L, Thomson ABR. Aging and the intestine. *World J Gastroenterol.* 2006;12(47):7578-7584. doi:10.3748/wjg.v12.i47.7578.

47 Perlmutter D. Choline is essential for brain development, memory, and even mood regulation. Yet, an estimated 90% of Americans fall short on this key nutrient. Instagram. Published June 2, 2025. Accessed April 16, 2026. https://www.instagram.com/reel/DKZqC-6t3Rw/; Zeisel SH, da Costa KA. Choline: an essential nutrient for public health. *Nutr Rev.* 2009;67(11):615-623. doi:10.1111/j.1753-4887.2009.00246.x.

48 Simopoulos AP. The importance of the ratio of omega-6/omega-3 essential fatty acids. *Biomed Pharmacother.* 2002;56(8):365-379. doi:10.1016/S0753-3322(02)00253-6.

49 Wu S, Ding Y, Wu F, Li R, Hou J, Mao P. Omega-3 fatty acids intake and risks of dementia and Alzheimer's disease: a meta-analysis. *Neurosci Biobehav Rev.* 2015;48:1-9. doi:10.1016/j.neubiorev.2014.11.008; Zhang Y, Chen J, Qiu J, Li Y, Wang J, Jiao J. Intakes of fish and polyunsaturated fatty acids and mild-to-severe cognitive impairment risks: a dose-response meta-analysis of 21 cohort studies. *Am J Clin Nutr.* 2016;103(2):330-340. doi:10.3945/ajcn.115.124081

50 Boardman HMP, Hartley L, Eisinga A, Main C, Roqué i Figuls M, Bonfill Cosp X, et al. Hormone therapy for preventing cardiovascular disease in post-menopausal women. *Cochrane Database Syst Rev.* 2015;(3):CD002229. doi:10.1002/14651858.CD002229.pub4.;Rosensweet D. *Happy Healthy Hormones: How to Rebalance Hormones and Feel Younger Again.* Institute of BioIdentical Medicine; 2017.; Bluming A, Tavris C. *Estrogen Matters: Why Taking Hormones in Menopause Can Improve Women's Well-Being and Lengthen Their Lives—Without Raising the Risk of Breast Cancer.* Revised and updated ed. Hachette Book Group; 2024.; Rouzier N. *How to Achieve Healthy Aging.* WorldLink Medical Publishing; 2007.

51 Sir Alexander Fleming discovered penicillin by accident. He certainly found something remarkable that he was not looking for.

52 Based on a Net Promoter Score of 67.

Made in United States
Orlando, FL
18 September 2026

87836195R10111